ATRESIA MICROTIA & YOUR CHILD

*HOW TO OVERCOME THE HEARING IMPAIRMENT
AND COSMETIC DEFORMITY CAUSED BY
CONGENITAL AURAL ATRESIA AND MICROTIA*

JOSEPH B. ROBERSON, JR., M.D.
HALEY M. ROBERSON, PA-C

The International Center for Atresia and Microtia Repair

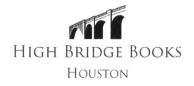

HIGH BRIDGE BOOKS
HOUSTON

Atresia Microtia and Your Child
by Joseph B. Roberson, Jr., M.D. and Haley M. Roberson, PA-C

Printed in the United States of America
ISBN (Paperback): 978-1-946615-70-1
ISBN (e-book): 978-1-946615-29-9

High Bridge Books titles may be purchased in bulk for educational, business, fundraising, or sales promotional use. For information, please contact High Bridge Books via www.HighBridgeBooks.com/contact.

Published in Houston, Texas by High Bridge Books

Contents

Dedication

This book is dedicated to the amazing parents of those children with CAAM who have entrusted me to care for their children—and those yet to come. The trust you have placed in me and my team is one of my life's most cherished compliments. This book is written in the spirit of bravely and honestly communicating treatment options while seeking to achieve the best results for your children.

And with special thanks and admiration to my oldest daughter, Caitlin Roberson, whose wordsmithing skills are amazing and have launched her professional career as well as improved this book immensely.

Letter to the Reader

Dear Reader,

As a young boy growing up in the mountains of Western North Carolina, one of my favorite times of year was late spring. During that time, my grandad let me accompany him as he prepared his fields for planting. He lived on a small farm and used a horse and plow. He depended on his crops for food and income.

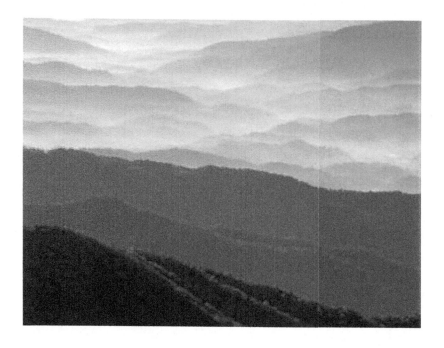

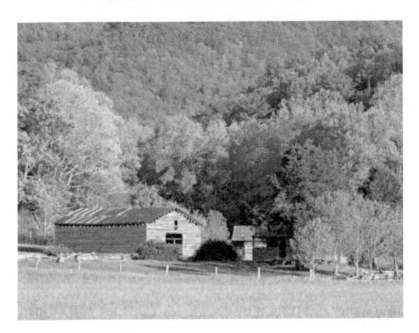

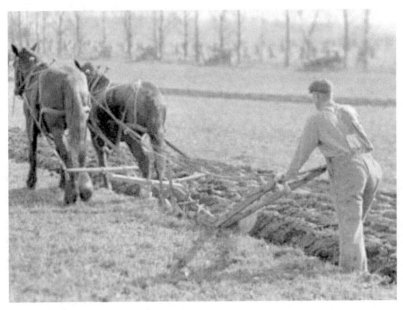

Mostly, I simply sat on the laboring horse as he walked behind me in the fresh earth, holding the handles of the plow. The sunshine was hot, and I watched as we went back and forth across his long, rectangular field. A barbed wire fence made of split wooden fence posts about 6 feet apart bordered the field. When it was time for me to help "man" the plow, Grandad would take me down from my perch on the horse to place his strong hands over mine and walk behind me, steering the blade through the soft warm earth. Our goal was to make grooves in the ground—called furrows—for seeds that would grow into his crop as the summer progressed.

Grandad taught me that the best way to plow a straight furrow was to aim at a fence post, keeping it firmly in view throughout the entire length of the field.

If I did not follow his advice, my furrow curved this way and that—creating chaos in the field (and re-plowing for Grandad!). Grandad had the love, wisdom, and presence of mind to teach me that **life is no different—seeing the finish from the start allows us to do our best without wasting effort or getting off track.**

If you want your child to hear, to speak, to listen, and to thrive in a hearing world despite the hearing impairment he or she was born with—or if you are gathering information about CAAM and its treatment options—this book is for you.

What Is CAAM?

Congenital Aural Atresia and Microtia (CAAM) is a physical ear abnormality that infants are born with. It affects the ear canal and the outer ear and is visible to other people. When these parts of one or both ears aren't developed, infants have hearing loss. If the condition isn't addressed, they will suffer developmental, social, and psychological effects their whole lives.

Atresia refers to an abnormal ear canal, and microtia refers to an abnormal outer ear. When these two conditions appear together, they are known as Congenital Aural Atresia and Microtia.

Due to the rarity of CAAM, few physicians understand the best treatment options, and correct information can be scarce. **Parents sometimes receive misleading advice given by people who aren't up to date on state-of-the-art treatment techniques for this rare condition.**

By reading this text, attending, or watching recorded proceedings of one of our conferences, you will access a knowledge base some parents don't have access to for years. Over the past two decades, we have made significant progress in the treatment of CAAM.

This thorough and succinct book will help you assemble the team that will overcome the effects of hearing impairment and cosmetic deformity from CAAM in your child's life.

The views expressed in this book result from my personal evaluation of and treatment recommendations for more than 5,000 children in more than 100 international conferences for parents with children who have CAAM; from many children evaluated at the International Center for Atresia & Microtia Repair in Palo Alto, California; and from surgeries I have personally performed on more than 3,000 children and adults with CAAM from more than 50 countries. The recommendations shared in this book have been strongly shaped by my experience as the father of three wonderful children.

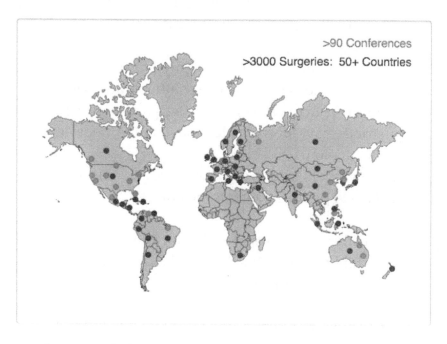

>90 Conferences
>3000 Surgeries: 50+ Countries

    I want to help you make a strong start as you begin to see what your child can be—as you begin to see your child's fence post—in short, seeing his or her end from the beginning.

With best wishes for success,
Joe Roberson, Jr., M.D.

This book could make a big difference in your child's life.

This book is for you if:

- Your child was born with CAAM
- You need help understanding and evaluating treatment options
- You want your child to hear, speak, listen, and thrive in a hearing world.

Due to the rarity of CAAM, many physicians are not up to date on the latest available solutions, and solid advice can be scarce. However, in the past two decades, huge strides have been made, and there is hope in almost all situations.

In this book, you'll gain knowledge some parents need years to gain. Its contents include:

- Different options available for helping your child have ears that hear and look as close to normal as possible
- How to evaluate those options
- Advice to assemble the team that will overcome the effects of hearing impairment and cosmetic deformity from CAAM

Please note this book gives general guidance only. Individual treatment plans need to be made by surgical specialists.

Introduction

Chapter At-A-Glance

This chapter includes:

A STORY: My experience as a parent caring for my own child with a severe condition and how this experience has shaped me as a doctor

DEFINITION: What CAAM actually is

SURGICAL DISRUPTION: When I first became aware of CAAM and developed the world's first all-in-one surgical procedure for the condition

INSTRUCTION: How to use this book, as well as its most important points

AN EXAMPLE: A letter from a woman who's had CAAM her entire life

Why I Approach Being a Doctor as a Dad

When I see children with hearing loss and look in their parents' eyes, I know exactly how they feel. Some are angry and frightened, while others feel helpless. Others are almost fierce in their insistence on hope. It doesn't matter which part of the world we're in—these universal emotions are natural parts of every parent's process when caring for children with critical needs.

I know because I've been in those parents' shoes.

A Newlywed, First-Time Dad, and Budding Surgeon

I fell in love with my wife, Julia, when we were both young. We married the week after I completed college, right before I started medical school. With a partner I adored and a deeply meaningful career, I didn't think my plate could get fuller.

I knew I was wrong when Julia shared we were pregnant. We became a family on June 7, 1985, when Caitlin Crist Roberson entered the world. I imagine every parent remembers the moment they first hold their newborn. Time was wonderful, and it seemed to fly.

The Day Things Changed

Twenty-eight months later, I was a surgeon-in-training in my ninth year of training after college. I loved interacting with patients. During this phase of training, I moved through different areas of surgery to complete my broad education before specializing in conditions of the ear. At that time, I served as a head of the emergency room (ER) and found it infinitely fascinating how many conditions our team of medical professionals seemed to be able to treat. Yes, the 24-hour shifts were grueling, but I had regular time off with Julia and Caitlin at least once a week. I loved those days. We'd go for hikes and stroller walks. Sometimes, we'd take my motorcycle to get ice cream. We lived on the third floor of married-student housing, and our second child was on the way. Life was exciting, demanding, and good.

One weekend, I felt sick after arriving home from one of my 24-hour shifts in the ER—likely from something I caught at the hospital. After vomiting, I opened the third-story floor-to-ceiling window in our tiny bathroom to air the room. I knew this wasn't safe for Caitlin, but Julia was suffering from severe pregnancy sickness, and I didn't want the smell to make her more sick.

The decision went against an agreement Julia and I had made several months before, when a friend of Caitlin's died of complications from falling out of a one-story window. I decided to tell Julia about the open window later since she was napping in our bedroom. Exhausted from work and from the virus, I fell asleep in the other room with Caitlin on my chest.

"She's Fallen Out the Window"

Several hours later, I jolted awake to the sound of Julia screaming Caitlin's name. While I slept, our daughter had run down the hall to see my wife while Julia was in the bathroom. (Julia hadn't yet put on her glasses and hadn't noticed the open window.) When Caitlin's socks encountered the linoleum, she slipped, and her body bumped through the exposed window screen.

As I ran to the bathroom, I already knew what I would see ... or rather, wouldn't.

"She's fallen out the window," Julia repeated over and over.

There Caitlin was, three stories down, lying unconscious on hard, clay ground.

I cannot describe the anguish I felt in that moment, nor how rapidly those first few moments passed. Before I knew it, I was down the staircase, around the building, and weeping as I held Caitlin in my arms.

"What are you doing?" Julia screamed, coming around the corner just behind me. "Why aren't you doing something?"

It was then that I realized Caitlin had literally just fallen.

From Dad to Daughter's Doctor

Looking at Caitlin's lifeless frame, for a moment, I was frozen. Was Caitlin still alive? If she was, had I paralyzed her if she had trauma to her spinal column when I picked her up?

"You've been trained to know what to do," Julia said—her intuitive wisdom as practical as it's always been. "Just do it."

The doctor in me took over.

"Call an ambulance," I said, checking her pulse. It was present but low. And Caitlin wasn't breathing.

Operating on automatic, I gave her mouth-to-mouth.

No response. Try again.

No response. Try again.

No response. Try again, heart sinking.

After agonizing moments, her breathing and heart rate began to return, but Caitlin couldn't breathe on her own without mouth-to-mouth for quite some time. We waited for what seemed like hours for the ambulance, and Caitlin remained unconscious. I continued giving her mouth-to-mouth.

Would the hours and hours I'd spent away from my family in the hospital save Caitlin?

A Patient in My Own Hospital

When we arrived at the hospital, we raced into the emergency room. What a role reversal. When I'd been there last, I was a doctor; everything was in order; and I felt in control.

The same IVs, lights, and beds were still there,
but everything else had changed.

One thing I knew—my family desperately needed my colleagues' help.

After evaluation in the ER trauma room, Caitlin was taken to the Intensive Care Unit on the second floor. Since Julia was so dehydrated from her sickness, she was admitted three floors above. I promised her, there on the fifth floor, that I'd do everything I could to make sure our daughter got the best care.

For the next blur of hours and days, I wandered between the second and fifth floors, sometimes with Julia, sometimes without. My main memory is the constant sensation that I'd walk through fire to help my daughter and wife. I was grateful for my colleagues, trained professionals who I knew I could trust.

It was an experience of the hospital process from the other side... and a lesson of what I'd intellectually known for years—having a loved one, especially a child, who is suffering produces the most excruciating emotions a human can have.

Integrating the Experience as a Doctor

I share this, dear reader, so you know that I speak to you as a surgeon-scientist *and* a dad.

Amazingly, miraculously, Caitlin not only survived but has since thrived—without lasting injury. While she's a happy, accomplished woman today, I will never forget what it was like to be her parent as we evaluated treatment options, made critical decisions, and navigated her healing process. Perhaps my keenest memory is how crucial communication with loved ones was, as well as simple explanations from the medical teams in times of severe stress.

I know what it's like to navigate traumatic situations and make life-altering decisions for your child. I know what it's like to crave information and advice. What treatment options are available? What is the likelihood of success? What are the different risks of different choices? Even for me—someone who "speaks medicine"—the choices were almost overwhelming. As I treat my patients now, I realize how critical accurate, respectful, and truthful communication is to parents with children in medical situations.

---

*I also know how invaluable it is to have the
partnership of trustworthy medical experts
who are motivated to do everything in their
power to treat your child.*

Understanding the Needs of Children with CAAM

Like other doctors, I first learned about CAAM during my residency in the late 1980s. In the 1990s, I noticed that many CAAM patients had serious problems in normal hearing situations, even after they received treatment. At first, I didn't think much of this. After all, correcting CAAM is one of the most difficult surgeries to complete. It's so hard, in fact, that many ear surgeons do not recommend the procedure to patients.

I'd learned through working with children needing cochlear implants that early intervention dramatically improved hearing and language results—especially in the first few months and years of life. As CAAM patients then received treatment typically between 10 and 12 years of age, I wondered if treatment timing was a contributing factor to the poor outcomes I observed.

At the time, CAAM treatment required a series of five or more separate surgeries. The first four surgeries corrected the appearance of the outer ear and caused a significant defect where cartilage was harvested from the chest to make the ear. The final surgery restored the missing ear canal. This sequence had never been varied.

During the early years of my career I was fortunate to treat a type of brain tumor that involves the hearing nerve. In the mid portion of my professional years, I was blessed to be involved in the early days of an implantable device that can bring hearing to deaf individuals called a Cochlear Implant. Needing a new challenge in 2003, I started the International Center for Atresia & Microtia Repair at Global Hearing, my organization, to develop better ways to treat CAAM. As you will see, different specialists are involved in evaluating and treating the condition. By bringing these experts together under one roof, I hoped we would collaborate to develop new and innovative solutions.

In 2004, I invited Dr. John Reinisch to speak at the hearing impairment conference that my team has hosted for 27 years now. We now do multiple conferences like this around the world each year (see atresiarepair.com for an up-to-date list). He spoke about a new technique he had developed for surgically correcting the outer ear. While listening, I realized an important thing—the ear canal could be surgically corrected *before* the outer ear was reconstructed using Dr. Reinisch's new technique. (Soon thereafter, I realized that these two separate surgeries might be conducted together *on the same day,* but we'll talk about that more later.) Dr. Reinisch confirmed that his portion of the procedure could be performed successfully regardless of whether the ear canal surgery was completed before or after his work on the outer ear. I began reconstructing the ear canals of CAAM patients *before* the outer ear surgery—for the first time in the world early in my career.

When I shared the success of the ear canal-first procedures in an article in 2009, this novel approach received opposition.[1] It disrupted existing methods and threatened to reduce the need for multiple procedures to a single surgery. Today, a decade later, the strategy has consistently demonstrated improved results in treating CAAM.

I'm happy to report we've seen a marked improvement in the hearing and language development of patients who undergo atresia repair when they're three to five years old.

Giving someone the gift of hearing—whether it's in one ear or both—is a huge deal. It proves to be a rewarding experience, and I understand that parents put profound trust in the doctors they choose to treat their children. Figuring out a treatment plan for your child's CAAM can feel overwhelming. This condition is almost always unexpected and discovered at birth. Parents face a new condition they, and sometimes their doctors, have never seen nor know much about, and accurate information can be hard to find. I intend to rectify that information gap in this book.

In the following pages, I'll help you clearly understand the choices and outcomes you have before you, and I will explain in frank and honest terms what I would do for my own child and why.

I hope you get to meet our incredible team members. I owe so much to the staff, care providers, physicians, and surgeons at Global Hearing who advance the art and science of treating this condition.

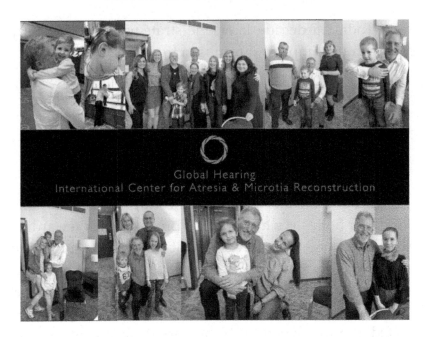

What Is CAAM?

Congenital aural atresia and microtia (CAAM) doesn't develop over time. It's an ear abnormality that is present from birth.

Definitions: Atresia, Microtia, and CAAM

Separately, Atresia refers to an abnormal ear canal, and Microtia refers to an abnormal outer ear. When these conditions appear together, they are known as Congenital Aural Atresia and Microtia (CAAM).

To understand CAAM, you need to know how hearing works in a normal ear. The outer ear focuses sound energy down the open ear canal. The tiny vibrations of sound cause a vibration in the eardrum—a delicate, thin, living tissue membrane at the end of the ear canal that separates the middle ear from the outside world with air on both sides. The vibrations of the eardrum are transferred to three middle ear bones, which act as a lever to amplify the sound energy and transfer that energy to the fluid-filled inner ear. The fluid of the inner ear receives the pressure wave, which enters the snail-shaped cochlea. In the cochlea, nerve endings are stimulated by the pressure wave brought by the middle ear bones, and electrical impulses are sent to the brain. These impulses are perceived and processed by the brain as sound.

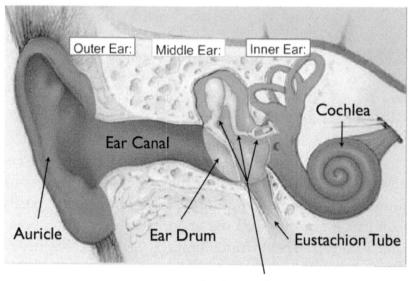

3 Middle Ear Bones

The anatomy of a normal hearing system: the outer ear (auricle), ear canal, ear drum, middle ear (containing the three middle ear bones), and the inner ear (consisting of the snail-shaped cochlea and hearing nerve, which transmits sound to the brain).

With **atresia**, infants can't hear normal sounds because they don't have a normal ear canal and eardrum. Bone occupies the space where the ear canal usually is, and the eardrum is missing.

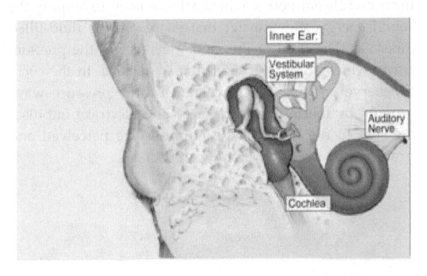

This image shows the ear of a child with atresia (missing ear canal and eardrum) and microtia (missing outer ear).

In almost all cases of atresia, children have middle ear bones, which you now know play a role in processing sound. However, the middle ear bones are usually partly malformed and fused to the abnormal surrounding bone, which prevents them from vibrating. Given the absence of the eardrum as well, the normal hearing structures are useless without intervention. Fortunately, the inner ear and the hearing nerve are almost always normal. In simple terms, it is often possible to restore hearing by surgically opening the ear canal, mobilizing the middle ear bones, and making an eardrum and/or by other treatment options summarized in this book that can bypass the lack of an ear canal/eardrum/middle ear bone system.

Children born with abnormal outer ears, or without any ears at all, have a condition called **microtia**. Because the outer ear is usually responsible for catching sound waves, this condition also contributes to hearing loss. How it looks can have significant social and psychological effects throughout children's lives. (Note: Aural Atresia and Microtia usually occur together. Atresia can occur as an isolated issue with a normal outer ear. Microtia, however, is always accompanied by abnormalities of the ear canal and never occurs alone.)

Many doctors don't realize atresia and microtia are related but separate conditions.

The options for microtia treatment (ear reconstruction) are straightforward. It's important to coordinate atresia repair, which is more complicated and requires much more specialized equipment and surgical techniques than microtia repair, when investigating one's choices for treatment. For the first time in history, our physicians have been able to combine surgical treatment on the same day for both conditions.

This Book's Important Points

If you're reading this book, chances are good that your child has CAAM. If that's the case, chances are also high that you're stressed, thinking about this often, and perhaps not sure what to do. You're probably worried about what to do while also determined to do whatever it takes to treat to your child. Therefore, this section summarizes this book's most important points.

On Emotional Care and Family Support

- **Talk with your family.** How are your emotions and heart doing? Dealing with a child's health issues can be hard, especially at first. Almost all parents are shocked when they learn their infant has CAAM, and the time and effort it takes to learn about the condition can be stressful. It is normal to experience varying degrees of anger, guilt, helplessness, denial, fear, sorrow, and grief.
- **Check in with your partner.** Parents move through their unique emotional journeys at different rates. Don't forget to check in with your partner and family members to see where they are in their journey.
- **Don't let emotions get the better of you.** While emotions are important to process, they also can impede timely decision-making. It's common for one parent to need longer than the other to process their reaction to their child's condition. In the case of CAAM, where waiting to treat the condition can impact the child's entire life, it's important to balance empathy and support with action.
- **Know this isn't your fault.** CAAM is generally not caused by either parent. While we'll

discuss possible causes for the condition later, know that this is not your fault.

On Evaluating Treatment Options

- **See the finish from the start.** You're about to face many important decisions. Knowing what you want for your child long term will help you be confident as you weigh different options.
- **Education is critical.** Parents who want their children with CAAM to hear, speak, and develop at the highest level possible must become knowledgeable about CAAM to make prompt decisions about treatment, therapy, and education.
- **Hearing matters more.** It is easy to focus on the way the ear looks. As your child grows up, however, the functional deficit of untreated hearing impairment is a bigger issue in the grand scheme of life. I have many adult CAAM patients who treated the cosmetic deformity of microtia but did not treat their hearing loss, and now they wish they had. Many didn't have the options we have today, others acted on poor information, but some simply ignored the problem.
- **Single sided CAAM will have severe hearing implications later in life.** We require two ears to develop and function normally (see later in the book). Since children can hear fairly well in quiet with single sided

CAAM in early years, some doctors tell parents not to worry about hearing. That advice is wrong.

- **Bilateral CAAM is a hearing emergency.** Children with CAAM in both ears (about 10% of patients worldwide) MUST have hearing treatment started within the first months following birth to allow normal development.

Do not overlook treatment for single-sided CAAM! The advice that "one-ear hearing is enough" is wrong.

On Making Decisions

- **The window to fix hearing loss is limited.** You must intervene and treat hearing loss in the first few years of life, or you miss the treatment window forever.
- **Act fast.** Timing is key to the successful treatment of CAAM—the earlier you seek treatment, the better.

Hearing loss will impact your child for his or her entire life if left untreated. This is the most important message to take from this book.

On Non-Family Relationships and Community Support

- **Connect with the CAAM community.**
  Along with talking to your partner, family,
  or friends about your emotions, it's good to
  connect with other parents too. Many of
  Global Hearing's patients and families are
  grateful for advice they received from others
  who walked the road ahead of them and
  shared experiences and advice. (You can
  find many support communities on the in-
  ternet, many of which occasionally meet in
  person. Please note this book does not neces-
  sarily espouse the advice given in these
  groups.) If you have the courage to reach
  out, you will be amazed at how much it can
  help you. The cycle may also repeat as you
  have the chance to help others.

The Most Important Points of All

- **Hearing loss is a disability. Normal hearing
  and brain function require two ears.** Early
  hearing—and in the case of hearing loss,
  hearing treatment—produces the best results. When treatment is delayed beyond the
  early years of life, the impact is lifelong and
  cannot be reversed with treatment at late
  ages.

- **The sooner your child gets treatment, the better.** Recent studies have shown another alarming phenomenon: Long-term hearing deficits may remain even after asymmetric hearing loss has been treated if the correction was not completed early in life within the "critical time window."[2]
- **Your child requires a personalized care plan.** While this book provides a framework for evaluation and education about the options for treatment, your child's hearing loss will require highly customized care to be effective. Since the anatomy of each child with CAAM varies, options for repair and success vary. Only a qualified specialist can help you create your own personal treatment plan.
- **Be confident in your child's future.** As hard as it may be to believe, there are worse things in life than CAAM. Treatment can be time-consuming, difficult, and expensive, but, ultimately, can lead to normal development without limitation for your child.
- **Communicate your confidence to your child.** While it is important to acknowledge and talk about your feelings, don't give your child a sense that CAAM limits them. When families honestly and courageously accept their situation and execute a timely treatment plan, their children can experience rich and uninhibited lives.

How to Use This Book

This book is intended to be a manual for parents of children with CAAM. It aggregates insights that my team has collected while evaluating more than 5,000 children at 100 international locations while performing more than 3,000 CAAM surgeries over the course of more than 20 years. You can read this book from start to finish in the order we wrote it. We also purposefully designed the content so you can skip from section to section as you need different information throughout your child's journey.

The first two chapters explain how normal hearing and language develop, and what goes awry in the case of a child with CAAM. The subsequent chapters explore testing and evaluation, treatment options, and results. These chapters follow a sequence I have refined and found maximally effective over many years of parent conference presentations and communication. If you are more of a visual learner, send us an email at atresiarepair@calear.com and we will give you access to a video of the latest CAAM lecture.

In the end, your child will need a customized treatment plan that requires consultation with a medical professional. By reading and understanding the information in this book, you will be prepared to understand your choices and determine the optimal plan of action for your child in consultation with a specialist.

Chapter in Review

- CAAM is a congenital birth defect that affects the outer ear and the ear canal.

- While hearing loss is a disability, there is hope.

- Normal hearing requires two ears.

"My Life Could Have Been So Different"

Global Hearing received this letter from a woman with single-sided CAAM, who we have not treated. She accurately describes some of the challenges she faces with the disability associated with single-sided hearing loss. I suggest you read it now. I will also prompt you to return to it later after you know more about CAAM. You will then understand why she had such difficulty in some hearing situations.

Dear Dr. Joe Roberson,

I just watched your video on microtia and atresia and am in tears. I've always felt so alone and almost crazy. After watching your video, I realize I'm not.

My life could have been so different.

At an early age, my mother suspected something was wrong and took me to many specialists. They all said she shouldn't worry—my hearing is fine; my left ear was just smaller than the right.

In school, I was constantly in trouble. When we read books out loud in class, each student continued where the previous reader left off. I was never able to do that.

I was told I was naughty. Teachers asked why I was not listening.

Children teased me and said I was dumb. I couldn't follow conversations, and I constantly asked what they were talking about. I did not know that I couldn't hear.

I started believing I was just not good enough.

I ended up hating school so much that I skipped almost every second day. In my last year, I started refusing to go. I studied at home and only went to school for exams. I completed school, not well, but I passed.

At some point in my adult life, I realized my hearing is not normal. I had it tested and found that I was deaf on the left side. I've been through a few operations to make the ear canal bigger. My third child was born with microtia and atresia of the left side [Note: This is very unusual as only a very small percentage of CAAM affects successive generations]. I was devastated. I felt responsible for him being this way.

Only now, at the age of 40, do I truly realize the profound impact my hearing impairment has had on my entire life. I look back and it breaks my heart.

I could have become so much more.

I still get anxious about being in a group of people, and I feel incompetent in conversations. Even though I'm now able to hear, it feels I'm lacking in cognitive ability. This has killed any chance I had of being confident.

I'm writing to thank you for educating people on the importance of hearing, especially from an early age. I have so many emotional scars from all that I endured. NO CHILD should ever have to go through this.

— A Mother with CAAM

Chapter 1

Hearing and Language Development

Chapter At-A-Glance

In this chapter, we will look at:

HEARING BASICS: What sound is and how hearing works

LANGUAGE FUNDAMENTALS: How children develop the ability to understand and use speech

HEARING LOSS: How hearing loss impacts children's entire lives

How Normal Hearing and Sound Work

Although they may be tiny, children's hearing systems are mighty. With the precision of finely tuned instruments, their ears capture and process sound waves—ultimately delivering them to their brains as electrical signals.

This section describes that process.

First, What Is Sound?

Sound is a complex vibration transmitted through the air. Imagine a stone being thrown into a pond. When the stone hits the water, a wave goes out in all directions. Sound operates similarly.

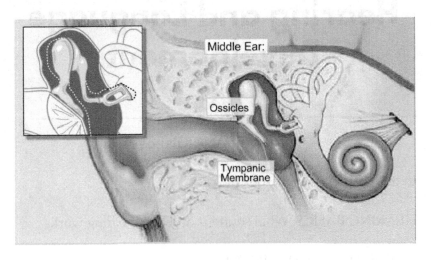

Sound enters the outer ear and travels down the ear canal. It then travels through the eardrum, making the ossicles vibrate in the middle ear.

How Does Sound Work?

When something makes a sound, vibrations travel away from the source in all directions. If people are in hearing range, their outer ears capture and send sound waves down their ear canals to their eardrums.

The Components of the Hearing System

The Ear and Ear Canal

The outer ear captures sound waves nearby and sends them down the ear canal.

The average hearing system captures more than 99.9% of the sound waves that enter the ear canal!

The Eardrum

The eardrum (or tympanic membrane in the graphic) is covered with skin. It has a middle layer of connective tissue and is covered inside with the same tissue that lines our nose and mouth, called mucosa. For hearing to work correctly, the thin tissue membrane needs air on both sides so that it can vibrate freely. When the sound wave strikes the eardrum, a tiny in-and-out vibration occurs.

Middle Ear Bones

The three middle ear bones (called ossicles in medical terminology) then transmit this vibration into the fluid-filled cochlea.

The Cochlea

The cochlea is filled with fluid and lined with tiny structures called nerve receptor **hair cells**. These cells look like little hairs and sway when sound vibrations make the fluid in the cochlea move. Think of these hair cells as thin blades of grass on the bottom of a pond. As the current moves, the grass sways to and fro. The movement of the hair cells makes them fire electrical impulses.

The Auditory Nerve

The auditory nerve receives the electrical signals from the hair cells and carries the electrical impulse generated by the nerve receptor cells to the brain.

The Brain

The brain is the hearing system's central processing center for incoming electrical signals, almost like a computer. Here, the electrical impulses are identified as sound and decoded to interpret their inherent meaning.

The entire hearing system is so tiny that the whole inner ear is filled with only a few drops of fluid. Surgeons must use microscopes to perform ear operations!

How Hearing Components Work Together to Create Sound

People normally think of the **outer ear** when they hear the word *ear*. The **ear canal** works like a tunnel, carrying sound from the outer ear to the **eardrum**. The eardrum passes sound vibrations to the **middle ear bones**, or **ossicles**, which deliver the sound vibrations to the **inner ear**. Called the **cochlea**, the inner ear is filled with fluid. It's responsible for converting the vibrations into electrical signals that the **brain** then interprets.

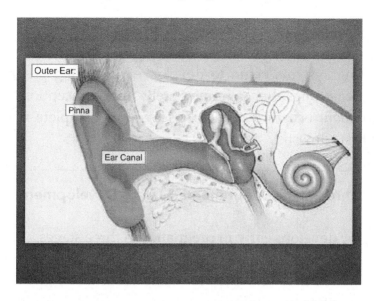

Normal anatomy of the human ear. Sound waves are transmitted through the ear canal, striking the ear drum, and are then transmitted to the inner ear (cochlea).

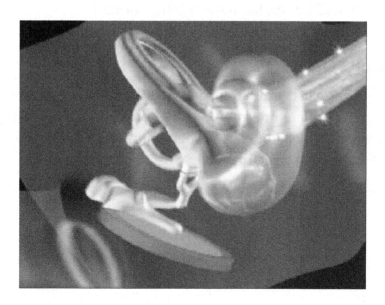

Vibrations entering the fluid-filled inner ear stimulate hair cells within the cochlea, triggering electrical signals which are carried by the hearing nerve to the brain, where they are interpreted as sound.

How the Hearing System Develops

Hearing systems begin to develop early during pregnancy—beginning almost immediately after conception. Development occurs in three phases and is complete within the first trimester.

Three Stages of Prenatal Hearing Development

The ear develops early in pregnancy in three stages.

1. The inner ear is nearly complete one month after conception.
2. The ear canal is formed before most women even know they're pregnant.
3. At 52 days, the outer ear has formed.

Stage 1: Inner Ear

The inner ear begins to form when the fetus is tiny and is nearly complete one month after conception. The cochlea starts off as a ball of cells. It then migrates to the skull base and forms that structure.

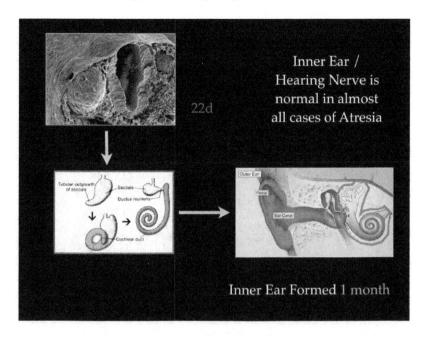

Inner ear development is completed within the first month of gestation. The development of these structures is typically normal in patients with CAAM.

Stage 2: Ear Canal

After the inner ear forms, the ear canal develops. It starts growing from the outside of the skull, where the ear canal is visible externally and grows toward the inner ear. A similar opening also grows from the back of the throat at the same time.

When the two tracts meet, the open ear canal is formed, with the eardrum in between. This process is complete before most women even know they're pregnant.

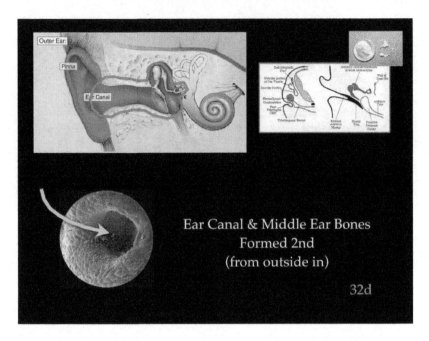

Ear Canal & Middle Ear Bones
Formed 2nd
(from outside in)

32d

Development of the ear canal and middle ear bones in a normal ear is completed within the first trimester of pregnancy. By definition, the development of these structures is always abnormal in patients with CAAM.

Stage 3: Outer Ear

The outer ear develops last. Six mounds of tissue form, grow, rotate, and fuse to make the outer ear. At 52 days, the outer ear is completely formed.

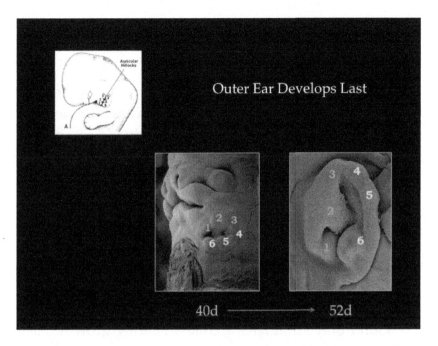

Development of the outer ear structures in utero. The outer ear develops last and is completely formed by two months after conception.

Can Children Hear During Pregnancy?

Yes. Babies hear in the womb and during birth. In both contexts, sound activates the ear, the auditory nerves, and the brain itself. In the absence of normal sound stimulation due to the hearing system abnormalities present in CAAM, the brain is not normally stimulated and, as a result, struggles to fully mature.

How Hearing Impacts Learning and Language Development

Your child's ability to speak, read, and write is inextricably linked to hearing normally. Without sound or hearing, speech does not develop as it can and should, even from before birth. Limited access to hearing and sound can also limit your child's capacity to read and write.

Studies show many adults with total hearing loss read at an average of elementary school level, likely because of limited access to sound! This is a sensitive topic for some individuals.

Sound only stimulates a child's hearing growth maximally for a limited period. If they miss this critical window, children lose the opportunity to develop normal hearing forever. The overwhelming majority of hearing and language development occurs within the first five years of life and is mostly complete by early teenage years.

Does Hearing Loss Hurt Brain Development?

Yes! The effects can be lifelong when a child's inner ear, auditory nerves, and brain aren't stimulated within the first months and years of life.

When these structures receive sound during pregnancy, infancy, and early childhood, they activate neural connections, both in number and size. Conversely, if sound is not accessed early in life, the number and size of neural connections are significantly reduced.

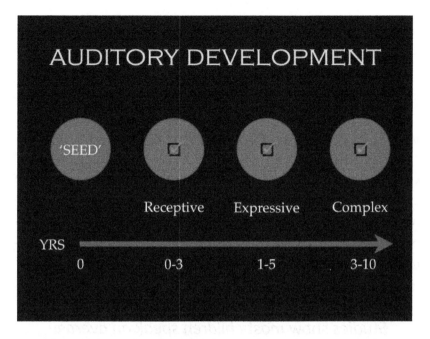

Stages of normal auditory development by age in years: receptive language (0-3 years), expressive language (1-5 years), and complex language (3-10 years).

How Children Learn to Speak

Normally, hearing children develop **receptive language** before they speak any words.

Receptive language is the ability to understand spoken words. It develops before children are able to say them.

When you learn a new language, it's often easier to understand than speak it, especially at first. Similarly, children understand words even before they themselves can talk. For example, when my children were about 12 months, they got excited when I asked if they wanted a cookie, even though they lacked the vocabulary to ask for one themselves.

The period of maximal receptive language development ranges from roughly from birth to three years of age.

When Do Children Develop the Ability to Speak?

Children generally enter their **expressive language** phase at about one or two years of age, and development typically lasts about five years. As long as their hearing systems process sound, a child's vocabulary quickly increases during this time, and their understanding of language structure develops.

Studies show most children speak an average of five words around their first birthday. By the time most are five years old, their vocabulary has blossomed to about 5,000 words.

With normal hearing, it's amazing how fast children develop!

When Is Hearing Development Complete?

The most **complex components of hearing** develop between 5 and 10 years of age and continue more slowly into the teenage years. Examples include directional hearing (the ability to locate where a sound is coming from) and hearing in noisy environments.

Sometimes, parents wait to treat hearing loss until too late—often because the effects of hearing loss don't show up until third or fourth grade, often due to poor school performance. At this point, treatment is usually too late because the critical period for brain and language development has already passed.

Effects of Untreated Hearing Loss

Common negative effects of hearing loss treated too late or not at all include poor comprehension in background noise, diminished learning capabilities, less-satisfying relationships, and smaller income—among other effects.

The Critical Speech Developmental Window

Even though hearing and language capabilities develop into teenage years, the most critical development period occurs in the first five years of life. While most of the relevant data has been collected from children treated with cochlear implants, the information still applies to hearing development in all children. In medical terms, this period is known as a **critical period of development**. Many body systems have critical periods of development similar to the hearing system. (I discuss this research in *Hear For Life: Dr. Joe's Guide To Your Child's Hearing Loss*.) As that book states (emphasis added):

> Hearing loss is treatable, and treatment may start at birth.
> It is extremely important to act quickly once the diagnosis of a child's hearing impairment is made or suspected.

If critical periods of development are missed, no amount of intervention can correct those losses. The age at which the treatment began is the single most important factor in predicting successful treatment of congenital hearing impairment in children.

In other words, if you don't treat your child's hearing loss within the first years of life, the damage can be irreversible. Do something as soon as you find out about it.

Chapter in Review

Sound is a vibration that spreads like the ripples in water.

The average hearing system captures over 99.9% of the sound waves that enter the ear canal.

Normal hearing systems develop within the first three months of pregnancy. Fetuses can hear even during pregnancy!

Hearing impacts language and speech development throughout the lifespan, especially in the first five to ten years of life.

Children who don't receive hearing in the first years of life may suffer the results their entire lives.

Hearing loss can impede overall brain development, as well as children's confidence, social abilities, and even income potential.

Chapter 2

What's Missing in CAAM?

Chapter At-A-Glance

In this chapter, we will explore:

PROBLEMS: Types and causes of CAAM

EFFECTS: How CAAM impacts hearing, language, and even brain development

IMPORTANT INFORMATION: Why humans need two ears, and why children with unilateral CAAM require treatment

HOPE: There is hope for children with CAAM!

Children with CAAM don't have normal hearing systems. No outer ear exists to focus sound down the ear canal. There is no eardrum. Bone completely fills the area where the ear canal normally should have developed and blocks sound from reaching the middle ear bones. This means children with CAAM can't hear normal sounds, like conversations, at a normal volume.

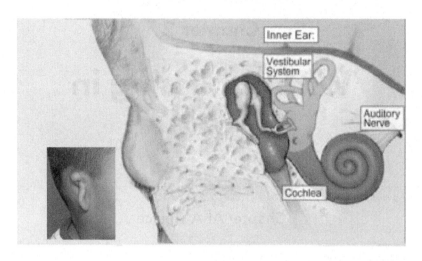

An example of anatomy in an CAAM ear. Note the absent ear canal, eardrum, and outer ear.

You may notice your child can hear louder sounds. This is possible when vibrations are loud enough to be transmitted through the bone of the skull, directly to the cochlea. Such loud sounds make it possible to test the function of a child's hearing nerves before CAAM surgery. At normal volumes, however, virtually no sound is received by or transmitted with CAAM.

Types of Hearing Loss

To understand this subject, I need to teach you a bit about hearing loss. Hearing impairment generally falls into three categories.

- **Sensorineural hearing loss** results from a hearing nerve abnormality.
- **Conductive hearing loss** indicates that either the outer ear, ear canal, eardrum, or

middle ear bones are dysfunctional. In other words, some problem with the outer or middle ear prevents sound waves from being conducted successfully into the inner ear.

- **Mixed hearing loss** incorporates both sensorineural and conductive components.

Types of CAAM

The kind of CAAM your child has will influence the best treatment.

- **Single-sided CAAM:** About 90% of CAAM cases affect only one ear. Ear abnormalities are more common on the right side than left. Infant boys also have the condition more often than girls.
- **Bilateral CAAM:** About 10% of CAAM cases affect both ears. In this situation, early exposure to sound via bone conduction hearing devices is a must. Without them, the hearing nerves and brain are not stimulated by sound, which prevents the development of normal speech and language and can severely and permanently impact the child's function over the lifespan.
- **Partial CAAM:** A partially formed ear canal and eardrum on one or both sides of the head occurs in a small percentage of cases. It's as if the ear canal and outer ear started to develop but stopped prior to completion.

- **Atresia only:** It is rare but possible for children to be born with normal outer ears but an abnormal or absent ear canal. When this specific condition does occur, it's likely due to a genetic disease.

Causes of CAAM

Almost every mother who has a child with CAAM asks herself if she did something during her pregnancy to cause the condition. Don't blame yourself or your spouse.

As far as doctors can tell, CAAM is almost never related to parents' actions or lack thereof.

We still have much to learn regarding the cause of CAAM. As we continue to learn more, I believe we will discover that genetics is responsible for most cases. The condition is, however, affected by more than just one abnormal gene. For example, I have treated nearly two dozen sets of identical twins, where only one infant has CAAM even though the twins share identical genetics. It is rare for both identical twins to have the same CAAM defect. If this condition was due to a single gene, both identical twins would always have the same CAAM defect since identical twins have an identical genetic makeup. In still other examples, in a small percentage of patients, we know CAAM is part of a larger genetic condition (medically called a **genetic syndrome**) that includes abnormalities of other body systems. Based on our current understanding of CAAM, genes are seemingly largely responsible for the condition, and some of these genes have been identified already.

By the time your children are having their own children, I believe we will be able to answer everyone's question: "What caused this and what's the chance my future children will have it?" Though doctors are making great strides in understanding leading indicators for CAAM, still much is unknown about the causes of the condition. Right now, we know the following:

- **CAAM is often independent of family history.** In the great majority of cases, CAAM affects families that lack any family history of ear abnormalities.
- **CAAM is sometimes associated with syndromes.** In a small percentage of cases, a genetic syndrome may cause the condition. We review such syndromes in Chapter 3.
- **CAAM does not tend to affect the same family twice.** Parents who have one child with CAAM rarely have a second. The rate of CAAM for later children goes up only slightly unless your family tree carries a gene that causes a syndrome specifically associated with CAAM.
- **CAAM is not usually hereditary.** Individuals with CAAM are only slightly more likely to pass the condition on to their children. The only exception is if a parent with CAAM also has a genetic syndrome; in that case, the incidence of CAAM is higher.

- **CAAM appears to be caused by a genetic susceptibility.** It may also be caused by another factor from the environment working together with a genetic susceptibility. A recent area of development called epigenetics may help unravel these questions.

How Hearing Systems are Impacted in Children with Single-Sided CAAM

In children with CAAM, the ear canal and the outer ear fail to develop normally. Whether present in only one or both ears, this abnormal development doesn't just impact the child's hearing system. His or her language and speech skills also suffer[3], as well as a variety of other factors that we will explore momentarily. Children with single-sided CAAM seem to function normally in quiet environments but have significant issues listening in normal environments.

CAAM's Impact on Language

Have you ever wondered why we have two ears? It's a good question to consider, especially if your child was born with single-sided CAAM and your family is trying to determine if one hearing ear is enough.

Our ears work as a pair.

Children and adults suffer limitations when they only have one working ear. Their learning and language are delayed. They may have trouble with social confidence because it is hard to hear in social settings. In this section, we'll explore why one ear is not enough—and how you need to understand that humans need two ears—before you make critical treatment decisions for your child with CAAM.

What Humans Can Do with Two Ears

When humans have two functioning ears, they have several distinct advantages over people who just have one working ear.

People with Two Ears Hear Different Signals

Each ear sends separate electrical signals to the brain. The brain uses these signals to perform important functions in our everyday lives that enable us to feel confident, stay safe, and make good decisions. Without two ears, children don't have access to important hearing abilities.

People with Two Ears Hear Sounds Louder

The same sound is louder when heard with two ears and is called binaural summation. Imagine someone calling you from another room. Two ears turn up the volume of soft remote sounds.

People with Two Ears Develop More Language

Language development is strongly associated with normal two-ear hearing. Language development is also strongly related to job and school performance.

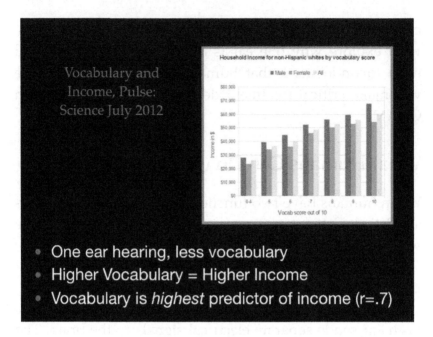

- One ear hearing, less vocabulary
- Higher Vocabulary = Higher Income
- Vocabulary is *highest* predictor of income (r=.7)

Hearing strongly affects vocabulary,
which is the strongest predictor of income.

People with Two Ears Tell Where Sounds Come From

Sound often reaches one ear faster than the other ear. Thanks to sound vibration inputs from both ears, our brains interpret the difference in timing to localize the sound source. This localization of sound is not possible with only one hearing ear. Normal-hearing people can tell where sounds come from without seeing the source. People with one ear have much more difficulty locating where a sound originated from.

Two Ears vs. One: A Practical Example

Imagine your child wants to cross a street. With one ear, she hears an ambulance siren. Unless she can actually see the ambulance, however, she can't know if it's safe to cross or if she should wait, because she cannot tell which direction the ambulance is coming from. With two ears, she can tell where the sound is coming from—whether it is approaching her or moving away—and determine her best course of action.

Children and adults with single-sided CAAM cannot localize where sound comes from. Furthermore, patients who wear bone conduction hearing devices (such as the BAHA, Ponto, or BoneBridge) likewise do not have directional hearing. We'll talk more about these devices in Chapter 4.

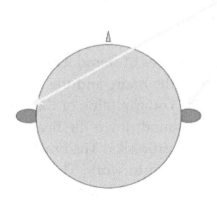

Being able to tell where sounds come from is an important safety skill, useful for many everyday situations, such as crossing the street or navigating a crowd.

Children without directional hearing visit the emergency room 20 times more often than other children.

In a less dire example, a child on a sports field might hear a teammate shouting, "Pass me the ball! I'm open!" Only with two ears can he or she know where the voice is coming from and respond.

People with Two Ears Hear Better in Noise

Almost always, patients who have had surgery to correct CAAM tell me they appreciate being able to understand sounds in noise the most. Why?

While individuals with single-sided CAAM hear normally in quiet environments, their understanding drops to 60% of capacity in moderate noise such as a busy meeting, restaurant, or classroom.

We spend most of our lives in a sea of sound. Our ears transmit the sounds around us to the brain, and the brain selects what we want to listen to. You can think of the ear as the receiver that sends every sound down the hearing nerve and the brain as the filter or processor. The brain requires two ears for the filter function to work. The brain also requires two ears during the critical period of development for the filter ability to develop—we are not born with it. Even people with two normal-hearing ears have more difficulty interpreting sound in loud environments, such as classrooms, crowds, grocery stores, the gym, or at coffee shops and restaurants.

Hearing in Restaurants: Can You Hear Me Now?

Imagine you're having dinner with a friend in a loud restaurant. Forks clink against plates; people talk at tables nearby; chairs scoot on the floor; cooks work in the kitchen; and so on. Even if you have two normal-hearing ears, you must work harder to hear your friend than you would in a quiet room, and it can be annoying to lose some of the conversation.

This same difficulty applies to other situations in public settings. Imagine how hard it would be to hear 6 of every 10 words your friend says! Imagine how that might affect your grades in school or your performance at work!

On average, a person with two normal-hearing ears understands 95% of words in background noise. Someone with a single hearing ear understands only 60-65%.

The above fact explains why children with single-sided CAAM are visibly frustrated, and sometimes distracted and/or disruptive, when classroom noise increases. They can't hear their peers or the teacher's instructions! Unfortunately, teachers often misunderstand this and think children have concentration or behavioral issues instead.

Given these challenges, it's no surprise that children with single-sided CAAM are 10 times more likely to repeat a grade in school, and adults with single-sided hearing loss earn only two-thirds of average income!

These situational and functional difficulties impact people with hearing loss for their entire lives.

What to Do When Doctors Say One Ear Is Enough

All over the world, I meet parents who have had a physician, plastic surgeon, pediatrician, or well-meaning advisor, say, "Your child hears normally from one ear. You don't need to worry about hearing or development if they have single-sided CAAM."

While one ear is definitely better than none, this reassurance is false—no matter how well-intended.

Such inaccurate advice is probably because, during training, most physicians don't receive education about hearing and language development. Now you know more than they do, and you can protect your child's future from irreversible developmental disabilities.

These well-intentioned professionals (and some parents) make the mistake of noting that a child's hearing performance in a quiet atmosphere appears normal, and, as a result, they conclude that no action is necessary. It is true that a child's performance in quiet with a single hearing ear does appear normal. The problem lies in the more difficult areas of hearing outlined above: directional hearing, soft sounds, and, most importantly, noisy situations.

It is important to understand this subtle principle: two-ear hearing must be restored to allow development of the capabilities listed above. Furthermore, hearing must be restored during the critical period of development, which occurs in the first few years of life. This period is frequently BEFORE the hearing impairments noted above are present since young children rarely demand much of their hearing in the first few years of life. **If left untreated, these limitations frequently emerge in the teenage years—at which time it may be too late to correct them, since your child is beyond the critical period of development.**

Success After Surgery Is Possible

Patients who have had restorative surgery for single-sided CAAM often tell my team that they can talk to their friends in the hall between classes for the first time. They also frequently report a dramatic improvement in how easily they understand new concepts in school.

Similarly, parents report that children hear for the first time from the car backseat, even while the radio is playing. They notice that they can call their child from a different room in the house, and, for the first time, the child knows where they are calling from. Others tell us their children hardly ever use the word "huh" anymore. Still more share that their child's grades have dramatically improved.

I shared a letter at the end of the introduction section where the writer describes struggling to hear in loud environments, and I told you I would prompt you to re-read it later. Now is the time to do that. It will give you a new understanding of how important this function is in a person's life.

Chapter in Review

Our ears work in pairs. Our brains cannot process sound at full capacity with input from only one ear.

Directional sound, or the ability to determine where a sound is coming from, is possible only with two hearing ears that are receiving independent sound input. Individuals with only one hearing ear, or hearing devices (such as the BAHA or Ponto) that stimulate both ears non-selectively, cannot achieve directional sound.

Normal-hearing people only hear at 95% capacity in noise. People with side-sided CAAM hear at around 60-65% capacity.

Often, teachers mistakenly assume that students with single-sided CAAM have behavioral or learning issues. In reality, the students' brains simply can't capture sounds in noisy classroom environments. Lack of attention, anger, refusal to participate and other similar behavior issues may emerge.

Common benefits that patients report, after they restore hearing in both ears, include better grades and more fulfilling relationships. Long-term statistics show individuals with two-ear hearing achieve higher incomes.

Chapter 3

Testing and Evaluation

Chapter At-A-Glance

This chapter examines:

HEAR MAPS: The world's now-standard framework for evaluating CAAM patients

BEST PRACTICES: How doctors should formulate treatment recommendations and how families can promote effective communication between medical professionals and treatment locations

---

It became apparent early in my work with CAAM that a standardized evaluation and classification system was needed for the condition to:

- Standardize the systematic evaluation of each patient
- Support efficient communication among medical professionals and treatment locations
- Promote accurate conclusions from treatment outcomes so we can better advise new patients on treatment plans

International Journal of Pediatric Otorhinolaryngology 77 (2013) 1551–1554

Contents lists available at SciVerse ScienceDirect

International Journal of Pediatric Otorhinolaryngology

journal homepage: www.elsevier.com/locate/ijporl

HEAR MAPS a classification for congenital microtia/atresia based on the evaluation of 742 patients

CrossMark

Joseph B. Roberson Jr.[a,*], Hernan Goldsztein[a], Ashley Balaker[a], Stephen A. Schendel[a], John F. Reinisch[b]

[a] California Ear Institute, 1900 University Avenue Suite 101, E Palo Alto, CA 94303, United States
[b] Cedars Sinai Medical Center, Department of Surgery, Division of Pediatric Plastic Surgery, Los Angeles, CA, United States

ARTICLE INFO

Article history:
Received 1 May 2013
Received in revised form 3 July 2013
Accepted 5 July 2013
Available online 7 August 2013

Keywords:
Otology
Congenital ear anomalies
Aural atresia
Microtia

ABSTRACT

Objective: Describe anatomical and radiological findings in 742 patients evaluated for congenital aural atresia and microtia by a multidisciplinary team.
Develop a new classification method to enhance multidisciplinary communication regarding patients with congenital aural atresia and microtia.
Methods: Retrospective chart review with descriptive analysis of findings arising from the evaluation of patients with congenital atresia and microtia between January 2008 and January 2012 at a multidisciplinary tertiary referral center.
Results: We developed a classification method based on the acronym HEAR MAPS (Hearing, Ear [microtia], Atresia grade, Remnant earlobe, Mandible development, Asymmetry of soft tissue, Paralysis of the facial nerve and Syndromes). We used this method to evaluate 742 consecutive congenital atresia and microtia patients between 2008 and January of 2012. Grade 3 microtia was the most common external ear malformation (76%). Pre-operative Jahrsdoerfer scale was 9 (19%), 8 (39%), 7 (19%), and 6 or less (22%). Twenty three percent of patients had varying degrees of hypoplasia of the mandible. Less than 10% of patients had an identified associated syndrome.
Conclusion: Patients with congenital aural atresia and microtia often require the intervention of audiology, otology, plastic surgery, craniofacial surgery and speech and language professionals to achieve optimal functional and esthetic reconstruction. Good communication between these disciplines is essential for coordination of care. We describe our use of a new classification method that efficiently describes the physical and radiologic findings in microtia/atresia patients to improve communication amongst care providers.

The article above[4] outlines such a system I put together with other team members called HEAR MAPS, which stands for:

- **Hearing:** Based on the results of the child's hearing test (audiogram), this measures the function of both the inner ear hearing nerve and the amount of hearing loss that the anatomical abnormality from CAAM has produced.

- **External Ear:** Describes the severity and type of outer ear malformation.

- **Atresia Score:** Based on a 10-point scale and determined from a special type of X-ray of the inner ear known as a CT scan. This score aids in determining candidacy for the surgical creation of an ear canal, as well as correlates with the expected hearing outcome after successful canal surgery.

- **Remnant Lobe:** Measures the amount of ear lobe tissue present.
- **Mandible:** Determines if the jaw bone is formed correctly or if it needs treatment too.
- **Asymmetry of Facial Soft Tissue:** Determines if the non-bone facial tissue is formed correctly or needs augmentation to look more symmetric.
- **Paralysis of Facial Nerve:** Determines if any abnormality is present in the muscular movements of the face, due to an abnormality of the facial nerve, which runs through the ear.
- **Syndromes**: Identifies any known gene abnormalities that are present which have caused CAAM and may cause other body system issues.

Every child should have an evaluation to determine every letter of the HEAR MAPS acronym to evaluate the best treatment options for their condition.

I also had a customized database created so we can track HEAR MAPS scores for every patient. This allows us to be scientific about our recommendations regarding what treatment works best for each combination of HEAR MAPS scores. The database now has more than 5,000 patients from around the world and serves to guide many of the recommendations you'll see in the rest of this book.

Let's take each section of HEAR MAPS separately and describe the process of evaluation. Our goal is to have a complete HEAR MAPS score to allow individually customized treatment planning. As you'll see, a complete HEAR MAPS score can be determined at 2.5 years of age or older.

Hearing (H)

Hearing tests are important for two major purposes. First, they allow us to determine whether the function of the inner ear, or hearing nerve, is normal. Second, certain types of tests allow us to quantify the amount of hearing loss caused by the outer ear and ear canal abnormalities present in CAAM. Both ears should be tested, whether or not each is affected by CAAM. In experienced centers, testing can be completed as early as a few hours after birth onward. Different tests are needed at different ages. This section is long and technical, so don't worry if you only skim it—you can rely on a professional adept at testing children to provide us with this data. I include it because it also outlines criteria to evaluate potential testing facilities and which tests you should make sure your child receives.

When Should My Child Get Tested?

Hearing evaluation can be performed within a few hours of birth. It is recommended that you test your child's hearing as close to birth as possible.

How Do I Find a Hearing Testing Center?

The earlier your child's hearing is tested, the better. This is the reason most states in the United States legally require hearing testing at birth. If your country or state does not provide this service, get on social media and ask other parents. You may need to travel to a major metropolitan area to find a facility.

If a facility hasn't tested children before, avoid it. If a facility doesn't employ someone who specializes in treating children, avoid it.

Where Should We Go for a Hearing Test?

Hearing can be tested at any age if the testing facility has the right objective testing equipment and personnel.

Hearing testing in young children requires experienced, highly trained, and talented pediatric audiologists and otologists, as well as expensive and delicate equipment. Many hearing centers lack the facilities, personnel, or equipment to conduct the required tests.

Because these test results are crucial for diagnosing and treating hearing impairment, it's essential to travel, if necessary, to a facility where such testing is performed on a routine basis.

What Data Should the Evaluation Process Cover?

As early in your child's life as possible, a hearing test needs to evaluate:

- **The health of the hearing nerve:** Typically, children with CAAM have a normally functioning hearing nerve.
- **The amount of hearing loss:** Children with CAAM generally have severe hearing loss from the ear canal abnormality. In the case of single-sided CAAM, it is also important to test the hearing of the unaffected ear.

Twenty-three percent of patients with single-sided CAAM that Global Hearing has evaluated also have abnormal hearing in the unaffected ear.

Fortunately, hearing loss in a non-affected ear can often be treated simply and quickly. Once a hearing impairment is suspected, the type and severity must be determined as soon as possible.

Categories of Hearing Tests

Your pediatric audiologist will use one or more of the following tests to determine if your child has a hearing impairment. In some cases, more than one test may be necessary to be 100% certain of the presence, type, and severity of the hearing impairment. Tests may be repeated several times to confirm the first test's findings, or to chart the course of progressive hearing impairment. Different tests may be needed at different ages.

Hearing tests fall into one of two categories. Briefly summarized below, we also explore them in the following sections.

1. **Subjective testing** relies on your child's behavioral responses to sound stimuli. Since subjective testing requires a participating, alert test subject, it's generally used with older children and adults.

2. **Objective testing** does not rely on your child's conscious expressive reaction. Instead, it measures electrical responses generated by the patient's hearing system and/or brain to determine if sound is being received and processed. As you may guess, young infants need objective testing. Because children must be soundly asleep and still for optimal results, this testing can be coordinated around nap time.

Sometimes, both types of tests are needed. Other times, just one is sufficient.

Your audiologist and otologist should be able to determine which kinds of tests your child needs. This is why it's important to trust your medical professionals!

Subjective Testing

Older children with some level of receptive language participate in subjective tests by raising their hands when they hear a beep. With younger children who cannot yet communicate, pediatric audiologists watch behavioral indications to determine which sounds children respond to. Examples include:

- Head turning
- Eyes widening to a sound
- A conditioned response that children show in response to other sources of stimulus, like seeing a toy

In general, children are old enough to accurately respond to a complete audiogram test when they are two to three years old.

Types of Subjective Tests

Several types of subjective tests exist for hearing impairment.

Audiogram

The most common type of subjective hearing test, an audiogram, determines both the status of the hearing nerve and what children hear in normal everyday situations.

A complete audiogram includes four tests:

- Bone conduction
- Air conduction
- Immittance
- Speech discrimination testing

Bone Conduction

Bone conduction measures the hearing nerve's ability to receive sound. (Impaired hearing nerves indicate hearing impairment.) Each ear is tested independently.

During the bone conduction test, a medical expert will place a device on your child's forehead or skull behind the ear. The device vibrates, and vibrations travel through the skull to the inner ear. If the inner ear nerve fibers receive and convert the vibrations into electrical impulses, the signals will continue to the brain and the child will respond. If the inner ear nerve fibers do not work, the child will not respond.

Air Conduction

Air conduction measures sounds heard through the ear canal. A medical expert will place a probe in or over your child's ear canal. The probe emits sounds at different levels of vibration and volume, and your audiologist will eventually be able to determine the softest noise that your child can detect at different frequencies.

Both ears are tested independently.

What If Bone and Air Conduction Tests Are Identical?

When your child's ears work properly, air and bone conduction tests will produce identical results. Inconsistencies between the two tests indicate where hearing impairment exists.

For example, when bone conduction results are better than air conduction results, a child most likely has a conductive hearing impairment. This condition is common in CAAM.

Immittance

Immittance tests use a probe in the ear canal. Obviously, this test works only for children with ear canals and eardrums. It is valuable for determining the cause of hearing loss in unaffected ears in the case of unilateral CAAM.

The test is quick and painless. It can be done even in young infants and even when patients are awake. A tiny loudspeaker emits sound waves, and an air pump generates varying the pressure in the ear canal. A microphone interprets responses.

By varying the pressure of the ear canal, it is possible to measure how sound bounces off the eardrum. The results indicate the status of the middle ear space.

- Normal middle ear space is only filled with air, which allows the eardrum to vibrate appropriately.
- Fluid or any other material in the middle ear space will constrain vibrations.
- In addition, the function of two small muscles attached to the middle ear bones can also be tested with the immittance probe. It provides information about the cause of certain types of conductive hearing impairments.

Immittance testing results are recorded in a graph called a **tympanogram**.

Speech Discrimination Testing

Speech discrimination tests are usually given to children and adults who have both receptive and expressive language. It goes without saying that it's difficult for infants to participate.

In such tests, a medical professional says a word, phrase, or sentence, and patients respond by repeating what they think they heard. Test results are evaluated by the accuracy of words and phonemes. (Phonemes are subcomponents of words.)

For example, suppose the audiologist says the word "rake," and the patient repeats the word "rate." That patient would receive a score of 0 in the word category because the word they repeated was incorrect. The patient would receive a score of 1 out of 2 possible points for phonemes because the patient accurately repeated the "ra" phoneme correctly.

Interpreting an Audiogram

Your audiologist and otologist can interpret your child's audiogram and should be able to explain the results to your family. This subsection is for parents who want to better understand how to read an audiogram.

The below image features the results of one child's audiogram. This child has CAAM. The numbers along the "y axis" on the left indicate the decibel (dB) level of sounds that child received during testing, more commonly known as the volume. The numbers along the top "x axis" of the diagram indicate the frequency of those sounds. The louder a sound needs to be for a child to hear it, the worse that child's hearing loss.

In this diagram, the line connecting the red triangles represents the hearing nerve's function, which is healthy and normal. The line connecting the green dots represents the level of the child's conductive hearing loss due to CAAM. The yellow dotted line represents where normal conversational speech generally occurs. The gap between the two lines is known as the "Air-Bone Gap," which signifies a conductive hearing loss. This type of loss can be mimicked in a normal ear by plugging the ear canal with a finger.

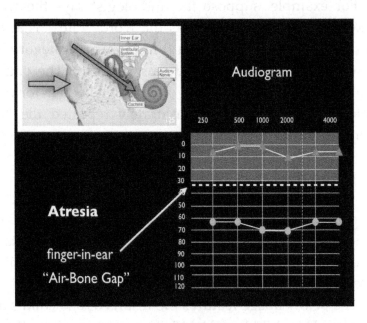

An example of air and bone conduction levels as depicted on an audiogram. The red line represents bone conduction levels, or hearing nerve function; the green line represents air conduction levels. The gap between the two lines indicates a conductive hearing loss, characteristic of CAAM. The yellow line represents hearing levels if the ear canal were plugged with a finger.

As you can see, this patient's ear only hears at volumes of 60 dB or louder, such as shouting. That means the patient does not hear normal conversational speech.

Conditioned Play Audiometry (CPA)

Conditioned Play Audiometry (CPA) utilizes the same basic testing parameters as a regular audiogram. However, an essential component of CPA testing involves conditioning a child to look at an interesting toy when a sound occurs. During conditioning, the toy generally uses motion and lights at the same time as a sound is made. Once the initial training is complete, the pediatric audiologist can tell when the child hears a sound by working in reverse. When the child expectantly turns to the toy, the tester plays a sound. If the child turns away from the toy toward the sound, this is confirmation that the child has heard the sound. CPA testing can generally be performed in children from 1 ½ to 2 years of age.

Objective Testing

Objective testing uses electrical or mechanical signals to confirm that the patient has heard a sound instead of conscious expressive feedback from patients during testing. This kind of testing is, therefore, suited for infants or other children too young to communicate what they hear, and when. It is also well-suited for patients who have other medical conditions, such as autism, that may prevent them from effectively participating in subjective testing.

How Does It Work?

In infants, the pediatric audiologist exclusively measures electrical responses generated by the patient's hearing system and/or brain to determine if sound is being received and processed. Infants must be soundly asleep and remain entirely motionless for optimal objective testing results to be determined. If not, muscle activity will produce electrical activity that can overwhelm the tiny signals coming from the brain's hearing signals.

For this reason, objective tests are generally coordinated around nap time and make use of over-the-counter medications that cause drowsiness, such as Benadryl. Sometimes sedation and even general anesthesia are required to complete objective testing.

Types of Objective Hearing Loss Tests

There are three most common types of objective hearing loss tests.

Auditory Brainstem Response (ABR)

An ABR is the most commonly used objective test for determining if hearing impairment is present. ABR tests produce results by generating several hundred broadband sound clicks and recording the responses. These responses sound like tic-tic-tic sounds. They are supplied to the ear with either a bone conduction device to test hearing nerve function or by air conduction in or over the ear canal.

Up to hundreds of clicks are released. As sound travels from the ear to the brain, the brainwaves can be measured by sensitive electrodes on the scalp and forehead. When sound is "heard," a waveform of standard configuration is produced. If no sound is "heard," no waveform is produced.

Because ABRs cannot provide as much specific information about each frequency as an audiogram, they are usually used to determine whether the hearing nerve functions normally.

Because the test measures tiny electrical impulses, and muscle movement of any kind generates electrical impulses, the test subject must be still during the test. This can only be accomplished during sleep or sedation for accurate results. In most cases, young children can have the test performed during a nap. Children who have trouble staying still will need sedation or sometimes general anesthesia for test accuracy.

Test duration is generally one to two hours and requires the pediatric audiologist to pick the correct waveforms.

Auditory Steady State Response

An Auditory Steady State Response (ASSR) examination uses some of the same equipment as an ABR examination. It is a newer technology that has been commercially available in the United States since it received FDA approval in 2001. Global Hearing provides ASSR tests instead of ABR tests because we believe the test is more effective.

Instead of presenting sound using broad or narrow band sound clicks, an ASSR varies its sound output, both in intensity and in slightly lower and higher frequencies simultaneously. A sophisticated computer analysis produces data records in a format similar to an audiogram like the one above—with more detailed results about specific frequencies of the hearing impairment.

Again, the ASSR test requires the subject to be still. ASSR testing can be performed faster than ABR testing, usually requiring one hour to complete. Not all centers currently have this technology available with adequately trained pediatric audiologists.

Oto-Acoustic Emissions (OAE)

As discussed, nerve receptor cells in the cochlea (also known as the hair cells) take the vibrational sound of energy traveling in the inner ear and turn it into electrical impulses. The hair cells transmit electrical energy to the auditory pathway, where it is carried into the brain for processing. As the hair cells receive and transform the vibrational energy, they have a tiny "twitch." The tiny hair cell twitches produce a miniscule sound—which is transmitted in reverse from the inner ear, through the middle ear bones, and back out to the eardrum—where it is released into the ear canal.

This type of testing can only be done when a normal ear canal and eardrum are present, so it's only used in the non-affected ear in CAAM patients. The sound produced by the tiny twitches is far too small to hear with our own ears. However, delicate instrumentation can detect and measure this sound.

Think of old submarine movies where the sonar man sends out a "ping" and waits for the sound to return. In a crude way, that's what the Otoacoustic Emissions (OAE) test does. Returning pings (or otoacoustic emissions) indicate twitching hair cells are present and active. As most sensorineural hearing impairment involves some disorder of hair cell function, this is extremely useful information. In a practical sense, if an otoacoustic emission is heard, we know the patient has hearing in the 0–25 dB range, considered within normal limits.

Several sources can cause inaccurate OAE test results. Fluid in the middle ear will overwhelm the sound generated by the tiny otoacoustic emission and can erroneously indicate an inner ear hearing impairment. Therefore, it is essential for this examination to be interpreted in light of other types of hearing tests by a qualified physician or audiologist.

Back to the "H" in HEAR MAPS

Two numbers accompany the "H." The first is the score of the hearing nerve function (also called bone conduction because of the way it is generated). The second is the score of air conduction testing using the following categories:

1. 0–19 dB
2. 20–29 dB
3. 30–39 dB
4. 40–49 dB
5. 50–59 dB
6. 60–69 dB
7. ≥70 dB

A person with normal hearing would be an H1.1, where both the hearing nerve and air conduction are normal. Someone with CAAM might have an H1.7, showing the hearing nerve is normal and the air conduction shows a severe decrease in hearing, which indicates a large conductive hearing loss. By using this shorthand method, we quickly document and communicate a patient's hearing status during our evaluation based on hearing tests previously performed.

It is easy to focus on the affected ear in unilateral CAAM situations. Don't, however, forget to test the other 'normal' ear! In our patient series, 23% of "normal" ears had a hearing loss. Since this is the only ear that provides hearing before treatment of the CAAM ear, it can have a big effect on how clear spoken language pronunciation becomes. If a small hearing loss is present in the normal ear, it must be known, as it affects the treatment plan.

External Ear (E)

When microtia is present, the formation of the outer ear (also called the pinna) can vary widely, from normal all the way to complete absence of the outer ear. For this reason, we categorize the amount of malformation as part of the evaluation process in the following categories:

- E1: Normal
- E2: Mild malformation
- E3: Moderate malformation
- E4: Severe malformation or absence of any outer ear

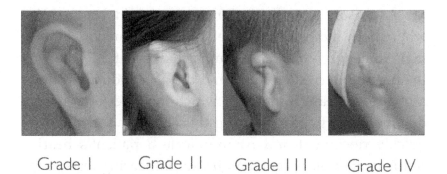

Grade I   Grade II   Grade III   Grade IV

Microtia is graded by the severity of the malformation into four types.

Most patients with CAAM have an E3 categorization of the microtia malformation. Patients who have an E1 and some patients with an E2 category do not require outer ear reconstruction.

In general, the more of the outer ear that is present, the higher the likelihood that a patient is a candidate for surgical creation of an ear canal. Of course, some exceptions exist.

Because the outer ear appearance does not guarantee the degree of formation of the middle ear (and due to other reasons you'll hear about further on), a CT scan *must* be performed to determine the potential for a surgically reconstructed ear canal. Some E4 patients will be candidates for ear canal surgery. Roughly 75% of E3 candidates are surgical candidates. A high percentage of E2 patients can have an ear canal if that path of treatment is chosen. However, it is impossible to determine if a patient is a candidate for certain treatments based on the outer ear appearance alone.

Atresia Score on CT (A)

CT scans are a special type of x-ray that allows us to see the middle and inner ear anatomy and determine the chance of success of making an ear canal. Scans are done when patients are still and take only a few minutes to complete. In small children, it's possible to complete scans at nap time, but depending on the activity level of your child, sedation may be required. **The earliest we recommend a CT scan is 2.5 years of age** to determine candidacy for the surgical correction of CAAM. In certain cases, your otologist may recommend a scan earlier in life if there are any specific concerns that need to be evaluated sooner. However, because the ear develops so rapidly in the first 2.5 years of life, we need to allow time for the ear structures to mature adequately before being able to use the CT scan to predict our chance of success with surgery. If scans are done earlier than 2.5 years of age, most commonly, it is necessary to repeat them at 2.5 years to evaluate the ear's anatomy and give a specific score to use in the HEAR MAPS evaluation protocol.

Computer algorithms render images that allow evaluation from different angles. In the ear, we can also use computer software to remove soft tissue and look at the bone.

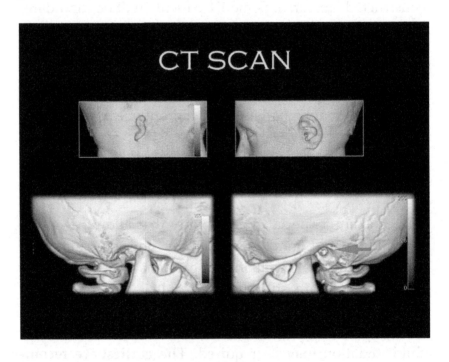

An example of a computer-generated model of a patient with right-sided CAAM. The red arrow indicates the presence of a normally-developed ear canal on the left side. In the opposite image, it is apparent that no ear canal has developed on right side, which is characteristic of CAAM.

The image above shows a three-year-old boy with right CAAM. At the red arrow, an ear canal exists on the left side as an opening in the bone. On the right side, however, no such opening is present.

Using the same data in a different way, we can change the image to view different photographic slices of the ear and surrounding structures, much like a loaf of bread is sliced. By looking at all the slices sequentially, surgeons get a picture of the 3D anatomy of the ear. In the following example from the same patient, bone is white, air is black, and tissue is grey.

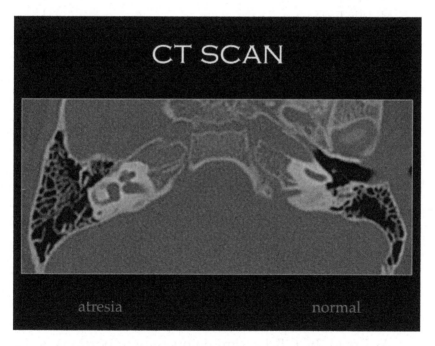

A CT scan showing a normal ear on the left (right side of the image) with visible canal, compared to complete atresia in the right ear (left side of the image).

When I look at such scans, I grade them with the following scale to give a numeric score from 1–10[5]. The higher the score, the better the chance of success. As you'll see later, the score of the scan estimates the likelihood of achieving a good hearing outcome if the ear canal were surgically corrected. Different parts of the anatomy get different points, and the total gives an overall score.

Atresia Score (Total Possible Points)	
Outer Ear	1
Middle Ear Space	1
Mastoid Development	1
Round Window	1
Oval Window	1
Stapes	2
Incus — Stapes Joint	1
Malleus — Incus Joint	1
Facial Nerve	1
Total Possible Score	**10**

It is important for the surgeon who is performing surgery to personally review the scan. I review every scan sent to us myself and won't perform surgery or even book a date for surgery before this has occurred.

As I read the CT, I assign points only to portions of the anatomy that are normal. On quick review above, you will see that an abnormality of the outer ear subtracts a point, so the highest most patients can score with CAAM is a 9. Later, I will share statistics on percent success with each score and how this data influences decisions about treatment planning.

In a small percentage of cases (about 4% of our patients evaluated worldwide), a tumor formed during a disordered development of the ears can be present as part of CAAM. This tumor will continue to grow and become life threatening to your child if left in place. Many physicians and plastic surgeons don't know this terribly important fact. Each year, I am referred patients from around the world where outer ears have been reconstructed over these tumors. The tumors are called **cholesteatomas**. The tumor grows slowly and usually silently, eroding into the bone of the base of the skull, and threatens or injures the patient later in life. These tumors can be identified on a CT scan.

If left untreated, a cholesteatoma grows and works its way into the inner ear, the facial nerve, or even into the brain. I'll discuss how to handle cholesteatoma in a few more pages. This is one of several reasons it is important to put together a team of professionals, so your child's short and long-term results are where we want them to be.

Cholesteatomas can be present with no outward sign. For this reason, all patients with CAAM must have a CT scan prior to any ear surgery or any kind – even if an ear canal will not be surgically created!

Lastly, the course of the facial nerve through the ear can be traced on quality CT scans. The surgeon performing a surgery for CAAM should study the CT scan to understand where the facial nerve runs. In rare cases, the facial nerve is in a position where it could be more easily damaged. Obviously, this is an anatomic detail that is best determined by the preoperative CT scan, instead of in the operating room during surgery

CT scan grading determines if a patient is a candidate for ear canal surgery and is the only way to detect potentially threatening conditions not visible on the outside of the malformed ear. Every child with CAAM needs one.

The patient's CT scan is the most important factor in determining if a canal surgery has a good chance of success. With CT scores of 6 or higher, canal surgery is recommended. Scores of 4 or less rarely justify the creation of an ear canal. Scores of 5 or on the border may make sense in some situations and not in others.

CANAL CANDIDACY

- Grading
  - < 5   Rarely Reconstruct (unless for HD)
  - 5   Reconstruct for some Bilateral
  - 6-7   Adequate chance of success
  - 8-10   Very Good chance of success
- Semi-Urgent Surgery
  - Cholesteatoma, some cases
  - Draining Ear and/ or Facial Paralysis

(Success Defined as Hearing Threshold 0-30 dB)

CT scan grade determines candidacy for surgery.

Interpretation and discussion of the CT scan findings with the surgeon of your choice are critical to success when considering whether to make an ear canal and eardrum to bring normal hearing to the ear.

In two situations, urgent surgery may be required. The first is for cholesteatoma, which is discussed further below. The second is for an uncontrolled middle ear infection in the atresia ear, which can spread to injure the facial nerve or to the brain, producing meningitis.

Remnant Ear Lobe (R)

The ear lobe is almost always present in CAAM. It is located abnormally—usually vertically—and displaced toward the face. Nonetheless, the earlobe is an important piece of tissue we use to make an earlobe in the normal position. Surgically, if possible, it is left attached but relocated to the correct position to match the opposite side. The amount of remnant lobe tissue is categorized in the following manner:

- R1: Normal
- R2: Reduced
- R3: Absent
- R4: Displaced

Mandible (M)

Mandible is the medical term for jaw. Twenty-three percent of the thousands of patients in our international database have an abnormality of the jaw associated with CAAM on the same side as the ear condition. The condition has been described as Hemi-Facial Microsomia (HFM).

Most patients with a jaw abnormality do not need treatment. As you see in the section on HFM below, some patients with severe jaw abnormalities do require reconstruction to lengthen the jaw. In the example below, a CT scan shows the left jaw, which is abnormal compared to the right. (This would be an M3 on the HEAR MAPS score.)

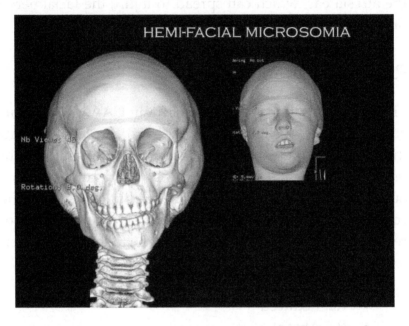

A CT scan reconstruction of hemifacial microsomia and underdevelopment of the left jaw relative to the right.

The M stands for mandible—the medical name for the jaw—and is described as follows:

- M1: Normal
- M2: Mildly reduced
- M3: Moderately reduced
- M4: Severely reduced or absent

Asymmetry of Facial Soft Tissue (A)

In a similar manner, the soft tissue of the face can be reduced in size on the side of the affected ear. This can be associated with a jaw abnormality (and usually is) but can also exist with normal jaw anatomy (an M1 above). To maximize the symmetry of the face and the appearance of the child, tissue augmentation can be done at the same time as an ear reconstruction. Most commonly, we remove fat from the abdomen with liposuction and transfer it to the cheek, where it fills out the deficiency and improves the symmetry of the face.

- A1: Normal
- A2: Mildly reduced
- A3: Moderately reduced
- A4: Severely reduced

Paralysis of Facial Nerve (P)

The facial nerve runs from the brain through the bone of the inner ear. It exits below and deep to the ear, where it runs through the salivary gland and out to the facial muscles. Each side has one nerve that runs to the muscles on the same side of the face.

Rarely, but importantly, the facial nerve function is abnormal as part of the malformation associated with CAAM. The facial nerve runs in an abnormal place compared to normal ears and needs to be evaluated carefully with a CT scan to determine safety of surgery[6]. The amount of movement when a child or adult smiles and blinks and moves other face muscles allows us to grade the amount of facial nerve function present. Reduced facial nerve function can mean an abnormal formation or position of the nerve and should be correlated closely with the CT scan to determine if surgery or some other treatment is advisable. An abnormal facial nerve function reduces, but does not rule out, the chance that an ear canal can be created.

We use the facial nerve scale developed by Drs. House and Brackmann, which originally described facial nerve function after certain tumors that can involve the facial nerve. We have adapted it for our purposes here:

- P1: Normal
- P2: Mildly reduced
- P3: Moderately reduced
- P4: Severely reduced
- P5: No movement, normal tone
- P6: Complete paralysis, no tone

Syndromes (S)

Lastly, we document if a known syndrome associated with CAAM is present. Please see the section on Genetic Testing below for further information on different syndromes. Our HEAR MAPS score documents if there is a syndrome and, if so, which is present. Patients with certain syndromes can have important needs and are even more rare than CAAM.

- S1: No syndrome
- S2: Syndrome present

An Example of One Patient's HEAR MAPS Score

Here is an example of a child with CAAM with his HEAR MAPS score.

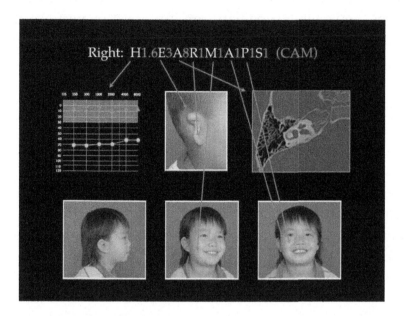

Right: H1.6E3A8R1M1A1P1S1 (CAM)

His parents chose to reconstruct his ear canal and outer ear at the same time with one surgery, called a Combined Atresia Microtia repair. (It is described fully below.) His hearing returned to the normal range.

Genetic Testing

Eight percent of our CAAM patients worldwide have an identifiable genetic syndrome. This percentage will increase as our ability to test genes improves.

All patients should have an initial general evaluation by their pediatrician. If all is normal, no further evaluation is recommended. If any abnormalities or questions come up in the first pediatric evaluation, a meticulous genetic evaluation by a specialist in Genetics or Developmental Pediatrics is needed. You can find these professionals in major medical centers, available by appointment. In some cases, your general pediatrician can assist or perform this service, especially if you live in a remote area away from large medical centers or universities.

Genetic testing is important to find other disorders—if they are present—that are beyond and sometimes more threatening than CAAM.

For example, the heart and kidneys can be affected in genetic syndromes that produce CAAM, and these conditions can remain silent until a serious problem surfaces if they aren't found early in a child's life. Evaluation by a specialist includes the following:

- A comprehensive physical exam
- Family history of medical conditions for the characteristic features of certain syndromes
- Tests such as scans and x-rays
  - In some patients, evaluation of genetic material is taken via cheek swab or blood test. Not all genes that cause CAAM can be identified … yet.

List of Genetic Syndromes

Here is a listing of genetic syndromes our team has evaluated that are most common among CAAM patients. Note that some are named for the scientist who discovered the condition:

Treacher Collins
Hemifacial Microsomia
Goldenhar
Chromosome 13 deletion
Crouzon
Pfeiffer
Apert
Nager/Miller
Oculo-Auricular-Vertebral
Klinfelter's
Klippel-Feil
Branchio-Oto-Renal
Pierre Robin
VACTERL Association
DiGeorge Syndrome (22q11.2 deletion)
Charge Syndrome
Chromosome 18q-
Chromosome 18 mosaic
Trisomy 13 (Down Syndrome)

Chapter in Review

HEAR MAPS standardizes CAAM evaluation and promotes effective diagnosis, treatment, and communication throughout your child's life, for your family, and for your child's team of medical professionals.

Hearing tests are important and should occur as soon after birth as possible to measure the health of the hearing nerve, the amount of hearing loss, and related syndromes.

It is important to evaluate the hearing status of both ears, whether or not they are affected by CAAM. Twenty-three percent of patients in Global Hearing's global database have hearing loss in the ear not affected by CAAM.

Chapter 4

Treatment

Chapter At-A-Glance

GETTING STARTED: When and how to begin treatment, including how to assemble a team of highly qualified medical professionals

THE HISTORY: A brief history of the medical treatment of CAAM

SURGERY & BEYOND: Best practices for preparation, healing, and recovery

---

When Should We Begin Treatment?

Determine your child's hearing loss as early as possible and begin treatment as soon as you can if conditions exist that can be corrected. The longer you wait, the more significantly hearing loss will affect your child's development. In in our conferences around the world, we recommend parents attend even if your child is a few weeks old. You begin to learn, and we begin to fill in the HEAR MAPS score and assemble a treatment plan. As your child is old enough to undergo tests, we'll be ready to plan treatment.

Usually, a CT scan at 2.5 years of age is the last test needed before finalizing treatment.

Assemble a Team of Medical Professionals

The first question to ask yourself is "Who do I need on my team to care for my child?" I suggest the following list:

CARE TEAM

- Pediatrician
  - *medical evaluation & well-child care*
- Hearing Testing Specialist (Audiologist)
  - *tests hearing and adjusts hearing devices prn*
- Otologist
  - *hearing decisions and auditory development*
- Plastic Surgeon
  - *reconstruct the outer ear (pinna)*
- +/- Craniofacial Surgeon
  - *jaw and facial reconstruction if needed*

A list of medical professionals to include in your child's "Care Team," as well as a brief description of their role.

Pediatrician

Your local pediatrician is a critical member of your child's team. She or he will act as your urgent, go-to person for most medical needs during childhood. He or she may also be able to evaluate your child for the presence of a syndrome. Your pediatrician will carry out the important well-care aspects that are important to ear health, such as immunizations and physical development tracking.

Hearing Test Specialist (Audiologist)

While a hearing testing specialist is called an audiologist in most countries, physicians perform similar functions in some countries. As outlined in the Testing & Evaluation section, different technologies are needed to give critical information about your child's hearing over time. A hearing test specialist will know what technologies are needed.

If a pediatric audiologist is available to you, get one on your team.

The pediatric audiologist's experience with hearing loss evaluation and treatment in childhood is extremely beneficial for our care of your child. In some cases, hearing devices will be needed, and pediatric audiologists tune and care for the devices that are used. As with your pediatrician, it is best to find a pediatric audiologist close to your home if possible, as regular visits are needed.

Otologist

An otologist (which is what I do) focuses his or her practice on the care of ear disease. A few even focus on the care of ear disease in childhood. The otologist is responsible for helping you interpret diagnostic tests after ordering them, evaluating your child's ear anatomy, interpreting CT scans, and performing surgery if needed. This person does not need to be local to you.

Plastic Surgeon

A plastic surgeon is responsible for the surgical correction of CAAM's outer ear deformity. Choose a plastic surgeon who specializes in the reconstruction technique, that I describe later, you prefer. Your plastic surgeon does not need to be located close to home.

Craniofacial Surgeon

In about 10% of all patients, a craniofacial surgeon is needed to coordinate and deliver care for the jaw and sometimes the facial abnormalities associated with CAAM or related syndromes. Craniofacial surgeons are specially trained in surgery of the mandible (or jaw), midface, and orthodontic or dental care. This person can live a long way from you if one is not available in your immediate area. Frequently, your craniofacial surgeon can work with local orthodontists if required.

First Steps

After parents assemble their team of medical professionals, the natural question to ask next is: "What do I need to do next?" I suggest the following **First Steps** action items:

FIRST STEPS

27%

- Hearing Testing
  - ‣ Hearing in the affected ear + "unaffected" ear

- Evaluation for Congenital Syndrome
  - ‣ atresiarepair.com - 12 Syndromes

- Speech and Language Dx / Rx
  - ‣ baseline allows follow up

- Early Consultation Otologist: Plan
- Surgical Candidacy: CT @ 2.5 yrs

A list of medical professionals to include in your child's "Care Team," as well as a brief description of their role.

As soon as possible after birth, a hearing test should be done to determine if the inner ear and hearing nerve in the CAAM ear is intact and functioning normally.

Remember, don't make the easy and tempting mistake of focusing only on the ear with CAAM.

In our experience, 23% of children with single-sided CAAM have hearing loss in their "good" ear.

If hearing loss is present on the side not affected by CAAM, serious implications on speech and language development are still possible. Fortunately, this hearing loss can usually be treated easily and quickly.

Through your pediatrician, a search for any of the syndromes known to cause CAAM is important. Many of these are identifiable at birth, but some may emerge later, and continuing follow up is important. If you are fortunate to be near a major medical center, a pediatrician may be available who specializes in identifying and treating genetic syndromes. Your pediatrician will know if such a local person exists. These specialists are called developmental pediatricians.

Beginning around one year of life, consultation with a speech pathologist may be a good idea. For example, if this is your first child, you are not used to what would be considered normal for a child's age. A speech pathologist can compare your child's speech and language development to that of other children their age. They may also be enlisted in your treatment team to perform speech therapy to help develop your child's vocabulary, speech, and sentence structure. In some settings, specialized schools adept at educating and developing speech in children with hearing loss are available and can be a phenomenal addition to your child's early life. Over time, our goal is to get hearing-impaired children enrolled and functioning normally in the school system. A speech pathologist will know what resources are available in your local area.

Within your child's first year of life, identify and develop a relationship with an otologist. This medical doctor will interpret and apply diagnostic information generated by pediatric audiologists and speech therapists and help you formulate a treatment plan. Also, if any skin tags or excess tissue or abnormalities need to be removed early after birth, he/she will perform this minor procedure for your child without disrupting any tissue options to be used later in the reconstruction process. Your otologist also can interpret CT scans and perform surgery.

By the time your child is about two-and-a-half years old, you should select an outer ear reconstruction option and add a plastic surgeon to the team. It helps a lot (and improves results) if the team members communicate well, are used to working together, and coordinate well as treatment is completed.

A Brief Historical Perspective of CAAM Treatment

A brief review of the history of the craft of treating CAAM may be useful as you begin to learn about surgical options.

Traditionally, microtia repair was performed using a rib graft technique and included three or four separate surgeries beginning between 5 and 7 years of age, after the ribs could grow to sufficient size to use in creating an outer ear. Using these techniques described decades ago, sections of three separate ribs were removed from the front of the chest wall and used to form a scaffold that mimicked the outer ear. The rib scaffold was then inserted under the skin to reconstruct the microtia defect. This process required several separate surgeries to complete and lasted over several years. After the rib graft microtia repair was completed, usually by about 10–12 years of age, ear canal surgery would then be performed.

As you read above, it is well known that stimulation of a sense during a critical period of development is crucial to the development of that sense—for example, the critical period of speech development described in Chapter 1. In the 1990s, I was the first surgeon to perform ear canal surgery before microtia repair. This change was pioneered to provide hearing to the developing brain and language centers of children with CAAM early in their life and developmental trajectory, at a time when maximal stimulation may occur. The new order of surgery challenged traditional medical practice at the time. In the early days, before I made this change, the average age of atresia repair was over 11.2 years of age—at which point the majority of the brain development associated with language has already passed.

We now perform hearing restoration surgery routinely at three years of age. The results on hearing and development are amazingly different.

My first publication of this work occurred in 2009 in several peer-reviewed medical journals. This change was directly facilitated by the development of the MEDPOR™ technique for microtia repair and reduced the total number of surgeries needed from four to two.

Our patients were happy with this reduction in the number of surgeries, travel, time away from home, psychological impact, and so on. I am so pleased young children can have restorative procedures without going through an operation more than four to six times. We have also seen improved language and speech and developmental progress in our youngest patients when hearing is achieved early in their life.

Several patients then asked if the Atresia and Microtia surgeries could be performed at one time. That polite and thoughtful question lead to an entirely new way to treat

CAAM. Today, we can complete the ear canal and outer ear procedures in one single surgery in some patients. Together, Dr. John Reinisch and I performed the first combined CAAM surgery in the world in January 2008. Today, I have completed hundreds of CAAM surgeries together with several surgeons. It is now commonplace for patients to select this combined option for CAAM repair.

Over the past 20 years, I have intentionally targeted the largest problems, complications, and limited outcomes for treatment of children and adults with CAAM. By doing so, we enjoy great progress in areas where results have been improved. I still have my original list from the beginning of the 21st century. The list is certainly shorter now, but we hope to make further improvements as we go along.

Surgical Options for Canal Surgery

As you have learned previously, patients with a CT scan score of 6–10 are typically best treated with the surgical creation of an ear canal. The flow diagram below will help guide treatment decisions. A temporal bone CT scan should be done at a minimum of 2.5 years of age, and not earlier, unless directed by a medical professional. While the inner ear and the middle ear bones are fully grown at birth, the bone around them grows rapidly over the first years of life and is not adequately developed to determine surgical candidacy until the child is 2.5 years old or greater. It is through this bone that an ear canal must be made. We must wait for the bone to form adequately before giving a score for the CT scan. We cannot use a CT scan at one year, for example, to determine the chance of success for surgery to make an ear canal because the bone through which the canal must pass is not yet sufficiently developed.

Note that grades 1–4 are best treated with implantable hearing devices, which are described further below. Scores of 5 can occasionally have canals created—such as in bilateral CAAM—but full hearing restoration may be less likely (but still helpful in certain patients).

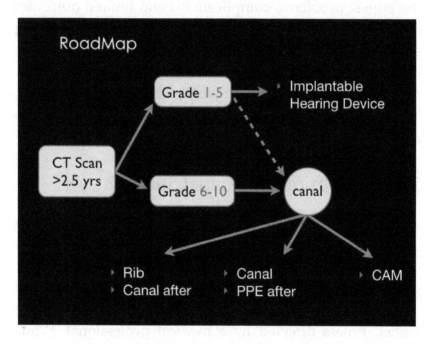

A road map to treatment plan options based on CT scan score.

Complex surgical equipment and facilities are needed to give a high chance of success. Surgical repair of CAAM is one of the most technically demanding surgeries that exists. The OR facilities require an excellent surgical microscope, special instrumentation, micro-drills, facial nerve monitors, laser, porous polyethylene microtia prostheses, in some cases customized middle ear bone replacement prostheses, and, in other cases, liposuction equipment. I cannot stress too much how important the correct equipment and staff is to the success of canal surgery. Since this is a challenging surgery, the ultimate results are achieved in operating rooms and by operating room teams who specialize in this surgery day after day, in the same facility with the same equipment.

Additionally, anesthesia for children undergoing surgery is a specialty in itself. I myself handpick anesthesiologists to staff our Surgery Center, and they are critical to the safety and success of the surgery. While most parents may not think of the large number of professionals needed to expertly perform these procedures, excellent team members are a critical component of success. As with any human endeavor, the world's best results are achieved when the same procedure is done time after time with the same focused team of experts working with the finest equipment in the same environment.

We operate under the guidelines that "if we would choose this equipment and this team to operate on our child, then we will do the same for your child."

The surgical equipment required to perform atresia repair surgery at the highest level includes:

- Facial Nerve Monitor: Electrodes are inserted into the muscles of the face after the patient is under anesthesia. Specially designed monitors are connected. Any stimulation of the facial nerve during surgery will result in a muscle twitch in the face. The muscle twitch is sensed and turned into an alarm sound to alert the surgeon and medical team, thus adding safety and protecting the facial nerve from injury.

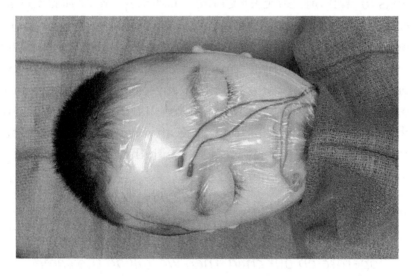

Facial nerve monitors in place, which are used to protect against injury to the nerve during surgery.

- Operating Microscope and Specialized Instrumentation, including lasers, submillimeter dermatome, and micro-drills

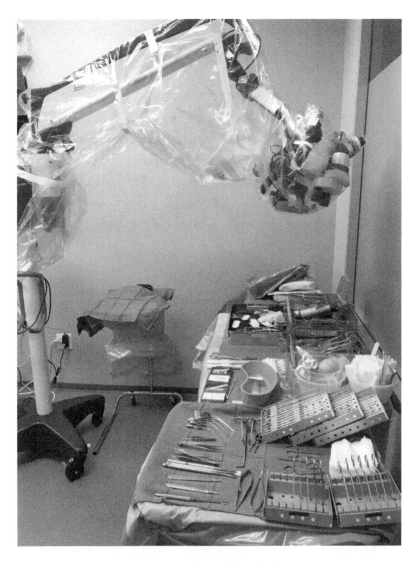

The operating microscope and numerous instruments required to perform successful CAAM surgery.

Canal Surgery Situations

As you will learn about below, ear canal surgery can occur in five situations:

1. When a normal outer ear is present with no ear canal or a partial ear canal
2. After rib graft microtia repair is complete
3. As a first step six months or more before separate microtia repair
4. At the same time as microtia repair with a Combined Atresia Microtia repair
5. Following PPE microtia repair. This combination is highly discouraged, as it puts the microtia repair at risk and should be done only in unusual situations.

The following are images of some of our patients who have had canal surgery:

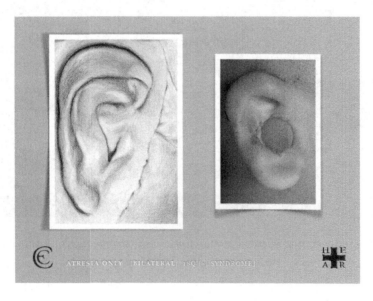

Scenario 1: Normal outer ear with surgically created ear canal.

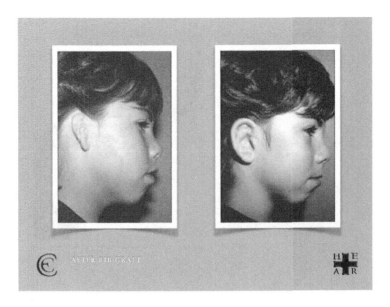

Scenario 2: Outer ear reconstruction by rib graft method completed prior to surgical creation of the canal in the correct position.

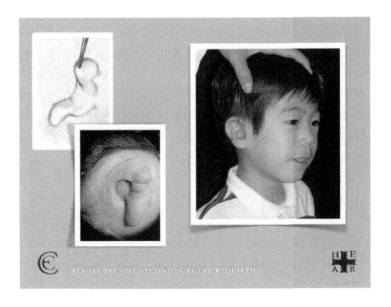

Scenario 3: Canal surgery is performed first, followed by secondary PPE microtia repair surgery a minimum of 6 months later.

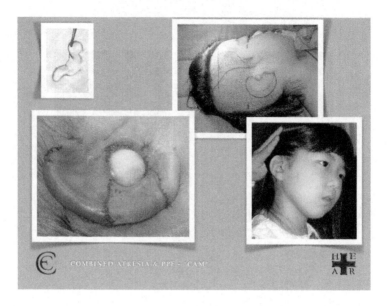

Scenario 4: Combined Atresia Microtia (CAM) repair, which entails creation of a canal and reconstruction of the outer ear with PPE in a single surgery.

Patients with adequate scores on CT scan are candidates for the creation of an ear canal. **Surgery can be performed as a separate procedure** (to be followed six months or more later by MEDPOR™ (PPE) microtia reconstruction) **or in a single combined surgery with PPE microtia reconstruction performed in one day**. Patients are discharged the same day as surgery in both cases.

Canalplasty

The surgery is performed under general anesthesia and requires approximately two hours for completion. Discharge takes place one to two hours after surgery. The ear canal is created in the normal position symmetric with the opposite ear in the case of unilateral CAAM. As you see in the images below, the new canal comes out just behind the small ear of microtia.

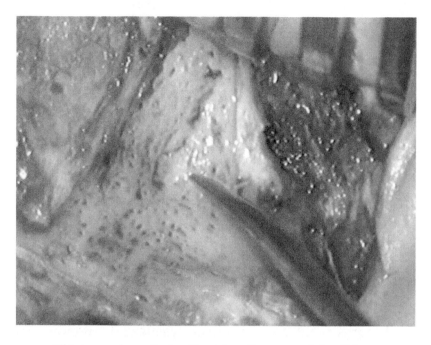

This image shows the location where the ear canal should have developed. In CAAM, this is instead solid bone, which is removed using specialized drills to create a canal.

During surgery, the abnormal bone present where the ear canal should have formed is removed using micro-drills and suction irrigation. Small diamond-tipped burrs of different sizes between 6 mm and 0.5 mm that rotate and sand away bone are used to sculpt the ear canal in the proper shape and direction. Continuous irrigation with saline solution removes the small bone chips and keeps the remaining tissues cool and healthy.

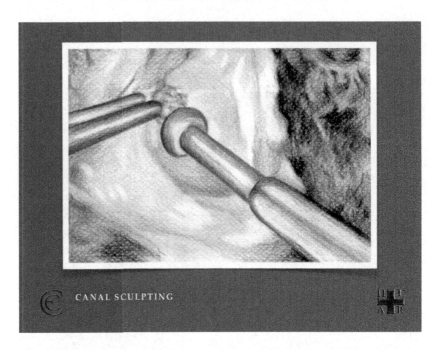

CANAL SCULPTING

Artist's illustration of a drill being used to sculpt the ear canal.

Progressively smaller burrs are used to remove the bone of the canal, stopping short of the middle ear bones, which are attached to the inner surface of the bone wall that is sculpted away to form the ear canal.

A laser is used to remove the last portions of the bony connection to the middle ear bones, freeing them to transmit sound vibrations for the first time.

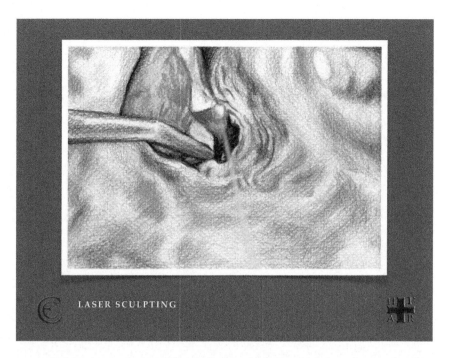

LASER SCULPTING

Artist's illustration of the laser being used to sculpt the native middle ear bones and free them to conduct sound vibrations.

After laser sculpting of the middle ear bones, they are checked to make sure they are mobile and formed adequately. If not, middle ear bone reconstruction using a custom prosthesis may be needed to bring hearing up to desired levels.

Since no eardrum is present, one must be created. A three-layered eardrum is fashioned, which mimics the same layers as a normal eardrum. The middle layer is a type of tissue called fascia, which is transplanted from the surface of the muscle above the ear and shaped to fit against the middle ear bones like a normal eardrum. Medial to the fascia, the body forms an inner layer of mucosal tissue during the healing process. Finally, the outermost layer is formed by part of the skin graft taken to line the newly constructed ear canal.

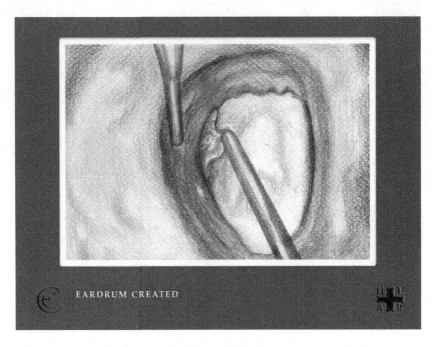

EARDRUM CREATED

An ear drum is created using fascia and secured to the middle ear bone chain in the appropriate position.

The ear canal is then lined with a split thickness skin graft that covers both the lateral surface of the newly transplanted eardrum and the surface of the newly created ear canal. Skin from the scalp has proven to be the most like normal skin, and the donor site heals without any scar. We have pioneered this donor site for skin in CAAM. A thin section of skin is removed, leaving the hair follicles intact in the scalp. The hair grows back on the scalp normally, and no hair grows on the skin transplanted to the ear canal.[7]

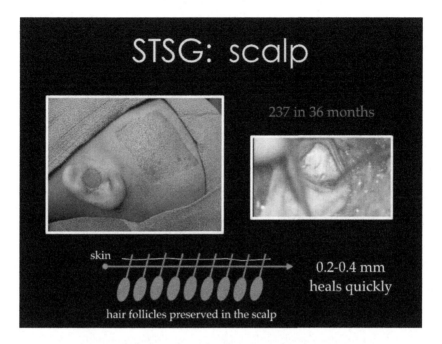

A split thickness skin graft (STSG) is harvested from the scalp, leaving the hair follicles intact, which will grow back through the graft site. The skin is used to line the newly created canal.

Packing is placed inside the ear canal that holds the eardrum and skin graft in position for two to three weeks as the body grows blood vessels into the transplanted tissue. The packing is removed at intervals in the postoperative period while the newly constructed hearing mechanism progressively heals. Between visits, we ask patients to place antibiotic drops on the packing at specified intervals, prevent water from entering the reconstructed ear canal, and to avoid high impact or jarring activity.

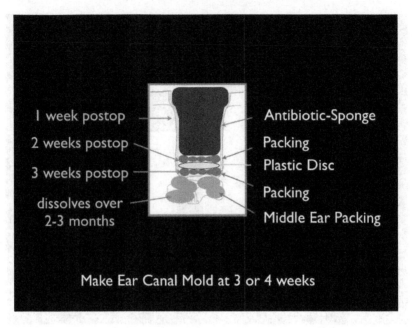

I week postop — Antibiotic-Sponge

2 weeks postop — Packing

3 weeks postop — Plastic Disc

dissolves over — Packing

2-3 months — Middle Ear Packing

Make Ear Canal Mold at 3 or 4 weeks

A graphic depicting the packing placed in the ear canal at the time of surgery, and a rough estimate of when it is removed in the postoperative period.

Combined Atresia Microtia Repair

Combined Atresia Microtia (CAM) Repair for CAAM is a single-step surgery where both defects of the ear canal and the outer ear are corrected in a single surgery.[8] An ear canal is created and the outer ear is reconstructed with an implant made of porous polyethylene (PPE), described below. Children should be three years of age and ~15 kg or more in weight. Two factors decide the earliest age we perform CAM surgery. The first is safety. General anesthesia is safest in children three years of age or older. As the procedure takes six to eight hours, anesthetic considerations for young children are paramount. We specifically use pediatric anesthesiologists familiar with the metabolism of the necessary medicines by children. Also, the amount of inhaled anesthetics is minimized by injecting local numbing agents (lidocaine and bupivacaine) both before the procedure begins and after it ends. As a result, patients feel no pain when they wake up.

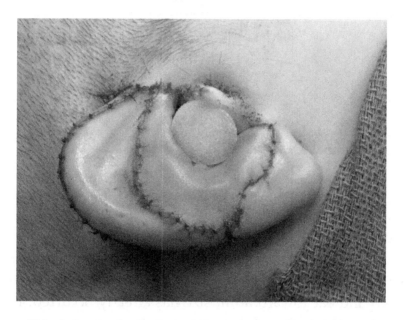

This photo was taken in the operating room immediately after completion of a right ear CAM repair. A protective silicone outer ear mold and head bandage are placed prior to the child waking up.

All CAMs performed at our institution have been accomplished as an outpatient procedure with same-day discharge. Because of our careful anesthesia processes, children can return home within a few short hours after surgery is complete.

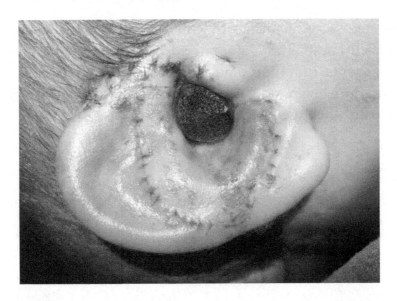

The same patient two weeks later. The outer ear mold and dressing have been removed, but the ear canal packing is still in place. The sponge in the ear canal will be removed at week three.

Coincidentally, 3 years of age is also a good age for surgery because a significant amount of growth of the head and ear toward adult size has already occurred. Figure 1 is illustrative of this growth pattern. As can be seen, the outer ear has reached 88% of adult size by 3 years of age and 92% of adult size by 7 years of age.[9]

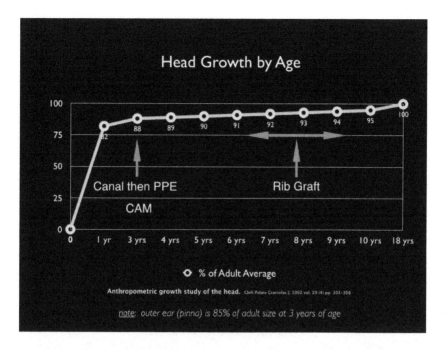

A graphical representation of head growth (percent of adult average size, y-axis) vs. age in years. By 3 years–the earliest age canal or CAM surgery can be performed – the structures of the head have reached 88% of average adult size. By age 7, they are 92% of adult average.

Both rib and PPE surgical techniques require implant size estimation based on anticipated final pinna size after growth has occurred by approximately 18 years of age. As such, the reconstructed ear and ear canal will appear slightly larger than the normal side in patients with unilateral CAAM. Later in life, when the structures have fully matured, both ears will match in appearance.

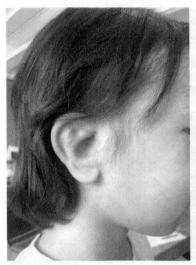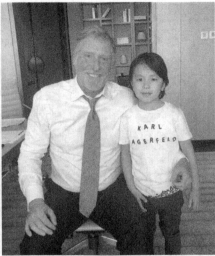

This boy is six months post-op after right CAM surgery and has hearing in the normal range (approximately ~90% of what a normal non-CAAM ear hears).

A frequent question is which technique of outer ear reconstruction gives the best hearing results. Hearing results following microtia repair using rib graft, PPE in CAM technique, and PPE in separate canal and microtia repair are identical. While hearing outcomes are the same, there are other risks and benefits that differ between these reconstructive approaches, which will be discussed in more detail later in the book. However, hearing outcomes are comparable between all reconstructive surgical approaches.

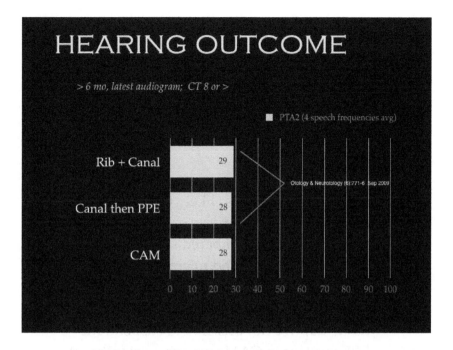

A comparison of hearing outcomes and reconstruction techniques. Note that there is no significant difference in hearing outcome between these techniques.

Microtia repair results utilizing PPE—whether implanted at the same time as canal surgery in CAM repair, as a second-stage procedure following initial canal surgery, or as a stand-alone surgery without ear canal creation—are nearly identical, with the following exception:

- Due to the ear being less mobile when a canal is in place, the PPE implant was more prone to fracture in the event of a strong blow to the ear in our early series. Still, overall fracture rates were low. Early results showed a fracture in just over 5% of patients. After instituting more significant welding of the connection points of the PPE scaffold, we believe we have this complication virtually eliminated, regardless of surgery approach.

Microtia repair results utilizing CAM repair differ from separate atresia repair and microtia repair surgery as follows:

- CAM patients are less likely to see the PPE scaffold become inferiorly or anteriorly displaced over time compared to patients who have atresia repair and microtia repair at different times. We believe this is due to the more vigorous suspension of the PPE with a tissue flap we can preserve to suspend the PPE implant in CAM surgery—a significantly stronger tissue than other suspension techniques applied in microtia repair following atresia repair. This tissue flap is not able to be used to suspend the PPE implant in a separate surgery approach, leading to slightly higher rates of implant displacement over time.
- CAM patients are less likely to experience canal stenosis than patients with separate surgeries.

In the operating room, an outer ear mold is made of soft material that hardens and is held in place with sutures. The blue outer ear mold stays in place for two weeks, and it cannot be taken off by children. Parents do not have to care for the mold in any way but must only keep their child from activities which might cause impact to or jostle the healing repair. The blue mold is removed in CAM patients ~2 weeks following surgery.

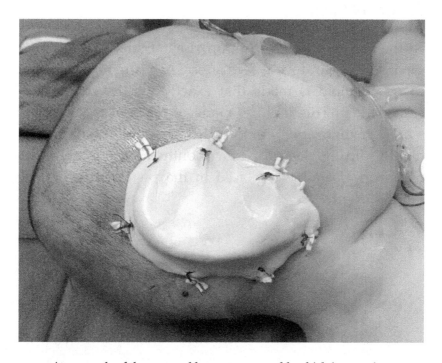

An example of the custom blue outer ear mold, which is sewn into place immediately after completion of a CAM procedure. This mold will stay in place for 2 weeks to protect the reconstructed ear before removal in clinic.

The opportunity for a "one and done" surgical procedure with CAM repair is extremely attractive to parents (and most patients!), especially to those traveling a long distance for services. A cooperative effort between pediatric plastic surgery, otology, and anesthesia is necessary to achieve excellent results in this complicated and long surgical procedure. To date, surgical results and complication rates in CAM are similar to or better than other forms of atresia and microtia repair. This makes CAM repair a good option for properly selected patients.

Ear Canal Mold

At the final post-op visit (approximately three weeks after canal surgery, or four weeks after CAM surgery), a custom ear canal mold is made that exactly fits the anatomy of each patient. This mold is made of material that reduces scar formation and promotes healing. The mold is used nightly during sleep for four months after surgery, with one drop of antibiotic placed in the ear canal before the mold is inserted.

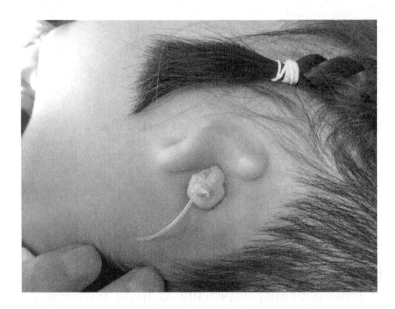

A custom blue mold is made for the patient's ear canal at the final postop appointment. Typically, this mold is worn for 4 months after creation, to prevent stenosis of the canal. If secondary outer ear surgery is performed after initial canal surgery, a new canal mold must also be made ~3 weeks after the outer ear reconstruction, to be worn for another 4 month period.

By using this mold in combination with exacting surgical techniques, we have been able to reduce the incidence of stenosis after canal surgery and CAM to under 2% of patients (compared to stenosis rates of approximately 20-30% worldwide). Use of the mold is critical to the long-term success of the repair and reduces the most common complication worldwide (stenosis) to a low level.

Complications of Surgery

Long and short-term complications occur in less than 10% of patients. These complications are typically treatable and require re-operation in less than 3% of patients.

Infection of the PPE implant is possible in the immediate postoperative period, but this has occurred in only two patients early on in our surgical series. A change to stronger intravenous antibiotic given at the start of surgery has eliminated PPE infections in the last 175+ patients. No case of ear canal infection has occurred.

In a normal hearing system, the eardrum is in direct contact with the middle ear bone chain, allowing direct transmission of incoming sound vibrations to the inner ear and brain. However, eardrum movement away from the ossicles (called lateralization) may occur late or early after surgery. Usually, pressure from the middle ear—such as otitis media—has been responsible. In the last several years, altered surgical techniques to secure the fascia graft used for tympanic membrane reconstruction has dropped this problem to just under 3% of patients. If hearing loss accompanies eardrum lateralization, revision surgery may be indicated.

Stenosis has been the largest and most common complication of atresia repair and may occur in up to 30% of patients worldwide. By implementing minimally traumatic surgical approaches, skin graft coverage of the bony canal, as well as other unique surgical techniques, we have been successful in markedly reducing this complication. Since 2012, the addition of a custom-made ear canal mold made three to four weeks post-op and worn for four months during sleep only (and discontinued thereafter) has reduced canal stenosis in our patients to under 2%.

Sensorineural hearing loss (e.g., damage to the hearing nerve) may occur with any ear surgery but has not been experienced in our CAM series. Similarly, facial nerve injury with resultant paresis or paralysis can occur from atresia repair. Worldwide, the risk of injury to the facial nerve is 1-2%. To date, my atresia patients have no cases of permanent facial nerve injury.

In dissecting the tissue flap used to cover the PPE outer ear implant, injury is possible to a small branch of the facial nerve that controls the muscles used to frown and raise the eyebrow on that side of the face. This is rare but can occur. Special care is taken in the operating room to monitor movement of the face and avoid permanent injury to the nerve.

Skin graft loss in the ear canal and or inadequate healing of the eardrum may also occur. Mucosal tissue may then instead grow and resurface on the ear canal, which may create a moist ear canal. Inadequate healing or lack of hygiene of the ear canal after healing can allow damaged skin to heal poorly in 2% of patients. Re-surfacing of the ear canal with a new skin graft and/or ear canal repair is needed in only a small percentage of patients. Most can be managed with topically applied preparations and treatment alone and do not require revision.

In this figure, worldwide complication rates based on published papers are compared to the complication rates in our patient series at Global Hearing (GHI).

COMPLICATIONS	Worldwide	GHI
Infection	2%	<1%
Eardrum Laterized	15-18%	3%
Re-Stenosis	20-30%	2%
Hearing Loss	2%	<1%
Facial Nerve Injury	2%	0%
Skin Graft Loss	15%	2%

A comparison of complication rates worldwide versus in our patients at Global Hearing (GHI).

Late complications may, of course, occur as well. These may require revision surgery at some point in a child's life. Revision rate curves with predictive analytics estimate approximately 10% of children will need revision surgery at some point in their lives. This may be due to a cause that would injure a normal eardrum (for example, a middle ear infection or wave striking the head during surfing) or a cause specific to canal repair surgery (such as lateralization of the eardrum or displacement of the PPE implant down-ward over the canal opening) among other rarer causes.

Cleaning the New Canal

Our skin constantly makes new cells and sheds old cells. On the outside of the body, these cells simply fall off or are washed away with baths and showers. In the ear, the cells can build up. Normal ear canal skin grows from the inside on the surface of the eardrum toward the outside of the ear canal. The normal ear canal is self-cleaning in most of us. When skin is transplanted from a different site as we use it in canalplasty or CAM, it does not migrate the way normal skin migrates. As a result, skin can build up in a recon-structed ear, forming a flaky coating on the canal and ear-drum. This build-up can block hearing and give germs a way to take hold and cause an infection.

During the first year following surgery, the ear will need to be cleaned by a local ear, nose, and throat doctor with a microscope (also called an otolaryngologist) two to four times. After the ear is fully healed, the cleaning inter-vals space out and finalize at one or two times per year for the remainder of a patient's life.

How to Prepare Your Child for Surgery

When it comes to recovering from surgery, children are much more resilient than most people think. Most of the time, it is harder on parents than on children!

I have found it to be important to communicate with children about approaching surgery. While detailed infor-mation isn't required, answering the questions of what they will feel and see before, during, and after surgery satisfies a child's naturally curious nature.

Here are some useful communication tips I've learned over the years:

General Communication Tips Before and After Surgery

- Give information to children at age-appropriate levels. For example, a three-year-old is satisfied with a brief description such as, "We are going to California, and Dr. Roberson will make your small ear look and hear like your other ear." Avoid too much technical detail. Older children may need more detailed explanations. You know your child and can judge how much to share, as well as how to share it.
- Answer any questions with brief and age-appropriate facts. This open attitude is a good way to reduce a child's concern in most situations.
- Avoid being secretive. Holding back can cause anxiety and distrust when your child inevitably figures out you have not been fully honest.
- Your child will not feel much, if any, pain just after surgery. This is due to the use of an injection of a numbing solution similar to what a dentist uses. This medication is injected before a child awakes from surgery. Later in the evening of surgery, the ear will

hurt mildly and can be controlled with pain
medication by mouth. There are no shots on
the day of surgery. Nothing hurts as your
child goes into the operating room.

- About half of children use pain medication
  the first night after surgery and then no
  more. The remainder of patients benefit
  from pain relief the day following surgery.
  Less than 5% of patients use any pain medication after that.

- Your child can read your level of anxiety or
  worry. Being confident and relaxed goes a
  long way with children as surgery approaches. Talk to your spouse or other
  adults about your anxiety and fear and remain strong and gently confident in front of
  your child.

Sample Conversation with a Young Child

"Mom and/or Dad will be there with you until you go into the
operating room to go to sleep. Dr. Roberson will be with you in
the operating room to take care of you while you sleep. We will
be there with you when you wake up."

[Note: we give a medication that sedates children and takes
away their memory of the 30 or so minutes before surgery so
they usually won't remember that portion of the day.]

Share Details about the Day of Surgery

- Your child will go to sleep by breathing from a mask similar to that of an astronaut or jet pilot.
- When your child wakes up, there will be a wrap around the ear and head. This needs to remain in place for a short time to keep them safe.

Advice for after the Day of Surgery

- Recovery occurs quickly over the first several days after surgery. Usually, parents are amazed at how fast children recover and begin acting normally. Most of the time you spend in California can be a wonderful family time.
- Mix your trip to California with a reward. Examples might include a trip to nearby locations, such as Yosemite, San Francisco, or Disneyland. The excitement of the upcoming adventure will focus your child (and you!) beyond the surgery. Traveling by car is easy, and our patients enjoy the many wonderful places they can visit in this state. It is also a time of togetherness for you with your child that may prove to be a wonderful time and memory.
- Keep a photo and/or print diary of your child's recovery. You can look back on it later and appreciate your journey. The remind-

er is also good for children as they recover and grow up; they will know how much you sacrificed to give them the gift of hearing. I have seen this appreciation grow throughout patients' lives, especially when they have their own children. The experience of being a parent themselves gives them a newfound understanding of how much you did for them at a tender time.

The effort you put into finding the best solution for this challenge is an act of love—and one that you deserve credit for going through.

Hearing Devices

Patients who are not candidates to have an ear canal created surgically or those who have had an ear canal created but need more hearing are treated with an alternative method of supplying sound to the hearing nerve. Our goal is to provide hearing to every ear. Once sound enters the inner ear of the affected ear, the electrical signal passes along the hearing nerve and enters the brain, just as it does in a normal ear.

Fortunately, a variety of devices are available to achieve this goal. In this section, I describe the important advantages and disadvantages of devices that Global Hearing uses, as well as how each works. Selecting the correct device is a complex decision and should involve your otologist. Frequently, more than one option is possible. This section is designed to augment, *not replace,* your discussions with your team of medical professionals about your child's best option or options.

New devices are always rapidly developing, and better devices will likely become available during your child's hopefully long and wonderful life. Different devices are available at different locations around the world. Technology that is now the best will not always be the best in the future, so try not to make decisions that make other wonderful options impossible later. It is important to choose technology from a stable company that is likely to exist during the entirety of your child's life.

Adopt a philosophy of "burn no bridges" when a hearing device is needed and selected. In other words, avoid any device which destroys the possibility of using other devices in the future.

How Hearing Devices Work

Hearing devices work in one of three ways:

- Bone Conduction
- Air Conduction
- Direct Stimulation

Bone Conduction Devices

Bone conduction devices involve external processors with a microphone and implanted portions connected to the bone of the skull. They turn sound into a vibration and transmit that vibration to the bone of the skull through the implanted portion. Bone vibration that happens anywhere on the skull travels to the cochlear and hearing nerves of *both* ears, where it produces an electrical signal.

Sound transmission to the skull bone occurs by one of three methods:

1. Direct contact of the vibrating device to a surgically implanted abutment.
2. By coupling the external device to a surgically implanted magnet with the skin intact in between.
3. By pressing the external device against the skull's skin with an elastic headband without an implanted portion.

Air Conduction Devices

Air conduction devices are the standard hearing aids worn by many with hearing loss. These devices need to be programmed in a slightly different way for children with CAAM, but they are the same type of devices worn by many older individuals with nerve (or sensorineural) hearing loss you learned about earlier in this book.

Air conduction hearing devices receive environmental sound, process it electronically, and augment it in a customized way for each patient. A tiny speaker in the ear canal then releases the processed sound into the ear canal at a volume louder than when it was received. Each sound is customized for each patient, similar to how a stereo equalizer makes sounds softer and louder, depending on what the listener finds pleasing and functional.

An ear canal must be present to use air conduction devices. When middle ear bone abnormalities prevent sound from improving to a normal level after canal surgery, air conduction hearing devices can bring sound up to a normal level.

Direct Stimulation Devices

Direct stimulation devices are surgically implanted hearing devices that apply a direct vibrating connection to the structures of the middle or inner ear, resulting in transmission of sound specifically to the ear in which they are surgically implanted. In current devices, an external speaker picks up sound and processes it electronically. The signal is transmitted across the skin to the inner implanted device which receives, decodes, and applies an electrical signal to a vibrating attachment to the middle ear bones or inner ear. These devices stimulate only the implanted ear.

Bone Conduction Hearing Devices

Cochlear BAHA Connect

Made by Cochlear Corporation from Australia, BAHA stands for Bone Anchored Hearing Aid. This product was the first brought to market and introduced in 1999 by EN-Tific of Sweden, which was then purchased by Cochlear Australia in 2005. It has been used for about three decades.

The device includes a surgically implanted titanium screw, which is surgically placed into the skull bone above and behind the ear. Attached to the implanted titanium device is an abutment, which comes through the skin and is hidden by the hair. It is a few millimeters in diameter and extends beyond the skin a few millimeters. The external processor clicks into the abutment and can be easily placed and removed for sleep or in the presence of water, which causes damage. With the external processor attached and fully operational, the device extends from the skin surface behind the ear approximately 20 millimeters.

Oticon Ponto

A nearly identical device first made by Oticon in 2006, the Ponto is an alternative to the BAHA Connect. It includes a similar implanted component to which the external processor is attached. Both the BAHA and the Ponto transmit sound vibrations to the skull bone, which travel to both inner ears as described above. These two devices compete regarding sound quality and additional features.

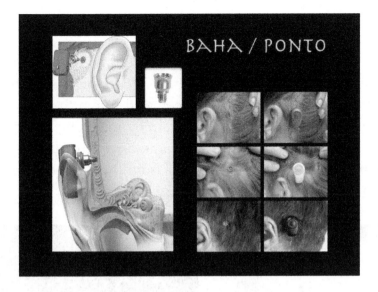

These images show examples of the BAHA Connect or Oticon Ponto, which includes a surgically implanted titanium screw that interacts with the external processor.

Soft Band (BAHA or Ponto)

With soft band devices, sound is transmitted to the inner ear by placing the identical processor used in the device's implantable version on an elastic headband instead. The headband holds the processor to the head. The device can stimulate hearing without a surgical procedure and can be fitted the same day a patient is seen.

Young patients and patients who don't want a surgical procedure frequently use this device. Others use it when waiting to institute other treatment types. Patients with bilateral CAAM should be fitted with this device within the first few months after birth. (See special conditions below.)

Cochlear BAHA Attract

This newer device (2013) couples vibration between the implanted portion and an external processor by the attraction of two magnets. Nothing comes through the skin. The device is held in place on the scalp by magnetic attraction. The external processor is the same as that of the BAHA Connect but projects out further from the scalp due to the magnet.

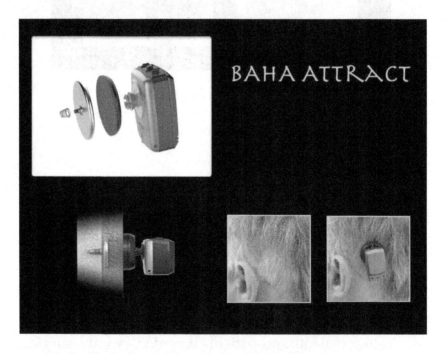

An image of the BAHA Attract, which includes a surgically implanted magnet that allows the external processor to be held on by magnetic attraction.

MedEl BoneBridge

MedEl Corporation of Austria first introduced a bone conduction hearing device in 2013 that implants the vibration-producing component under the skin. (The devices above leave the vibration-producing portion outside the body.) Nothing comes through the skin.

A magnet holds an external processor in place, which includes the microphone, battery, and software. The external device transmits sound across the skin to the internal device. The vibrating portion of the device is 9 mm thick and can be difficult to place in young children, as their skull thickness is less than 5 mm at five years of age. While some surgeons move the device down to the thicker bone of the lower skull, called the mastoid, this placement can interfere with placement of the microtia repair implant (either rib or PPE). As such, this device may be best reserved for adults. The device is not FDA approved and therefore not available in the USA.

Air Conduction Hearing Devices

Multiple manufacturers produce air conduction hearing devices. The worldwide market is close to 7 billion U.S. dollars. They fit the ear canal with custom molds and do not require surgery. Varieties exist for placement in the canal, in the ear, or behind the ear. They are used when awake and must be removed in a wet environment. Batteries are required every few days to power them.

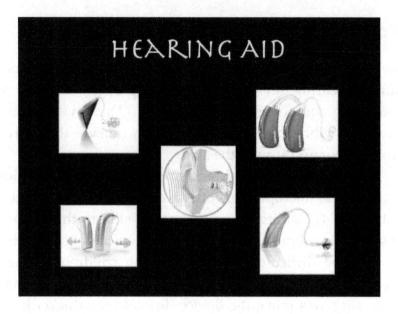

Examples of air conduction hearing aids, which can amplify incoming sound in the presence of an ear canal and boost hearing levels.

Many choices of hearing aids exist, and the device best suited for each patient is determined by an audiologist specializing in hearing aid fittings. For children, pediatric audiologists are the best choice for seeking advice.

In some varieties, the device is held in place by the outer ear. With rib graft implants, the groove behind the ear typically is not present, and these devices must be held on with double-sided tape. In patients with PPE implants, the device must not push on the skin overlying the implant, as it may lead to skin injury and PPE implant problems. Both precautions are handled easily with a few tips from your audiologist.

Direct Stimulation Devices

MedEl Vibrant SoundBridge

MedEl offers another device for hearing restoration in a small number of patients. The implanted portion is situated under the skin above and behind the ear. An external processor picks up sound and passes it to the internal device. The two are held together by magnetic attraction. No part of the device comes through the skin.

The internal implant behind the ear is connected by a thin wire to an additional vibrating component about twice the size of a grain of rice. This component, called the floating mass transducer, can be surgically placed in the middle ear and attached to a middle ear bone, or to a part of the ear where sound is transmitted.[10] The vibrations generated by the transducer are directly transmitted through the hearing system and on to the brain.

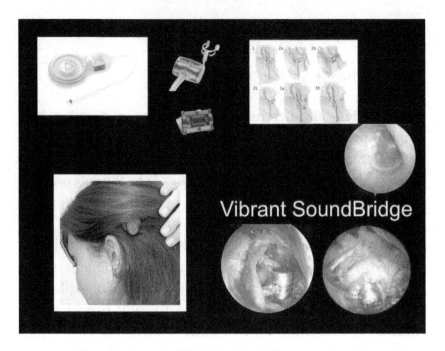

Images of the MedEl Vibrant SoundBridge implantable device.

As an interesting side note, the inventor of the Vibrant SoundBridge device has hearing loss and himself received implantation with this device. The images you see in the bottom right are actual photos of his device when it was surgically placed. He and I worked together when I was in training at Stanford University, in the hearing research facility where he first invented this device. Years later, I did the surgery for him, which was when these pictures were taken.

Disadvantages of Bone Conduction Hearing Aids (BCHAs)

Stimulation with a bone conduction hearing aid (BAHA, Ponto, Sophono, BoneBridge) stimulates both inner ears with the same signal. Since the brain needs two separate data streams to localize sounds, a bone conduction hearing aid does not provide the information needed for the brain to perform this function. Bone conduction hearing aids do not allow patients to localize sound even if two are worn.

Likewise, since the brain needs two ear data streams to hear normally in background noise, and since BCHAs do not provide it, hearing in noise with BCHAs is not ideal. BCHAs are most helpful in low to moderate noise situations. We have seen repeatedly that children with unilateral CAAM who wear a BCHA voluntarily remove these devices in moderate to high noise situations. The reason is the good ear—the non-CAAM ear—is getting sound from both the normal ear canal and hearing mechanism AND from the BCHA. When sound environments get louder, the two sounds together are confusing, and patients hear with only the normal hearing ear.

The sound quality of implanted bone conduction devices is also somewhat synthetic. Patients describe the sound as robotic or machine-like with a higher-than-normal high-frequency component. The sound is, however, functional and useful for both speech understanding and development.

If a bone conduction device is the best choice for you or your child, you should be clear that revision surgery will be needed in almost 100% of pediatric patients. This is rarely shared by surgeons recommending these devices. Two sources cause the need for revision:

- Infection and/or the device coming out. In BCHA devices with a component through the skin (such as the BAHA Connect or Oticon Ponto), local skin infection occurs an average of 2.3 times per year. These are typically easily treatable with gentle cleaning and topical medications but may require revision.

- Extrusion of implantable bone conduction hearing devices happens in 8% of patients. This means the inserted portion of the device will come out.

- As a child grows, both the skin of the scalp and the thickness of the skull increase significantly. (For example, children around five years of age have a skull skin thickness of 4-5 mm and adults have a skull skin thickness of 12-17 mm.) Due to these changes, there is nearly a 100% chance a portion of the implant will need to be changed when a child becomes an adult.

The cost of implantable BCHAs may be less than surgery for an ear canal at first. In the long run, the cost of implantable devices is significantly more. External processors are replaced on average every four to five years for life, and each replacement is $5,000–7,000 in U.S. dollars. Revision surgery is inevitable and will also add a financial burden.

Patients with bilateral CAAM should be fitted with bone conduction hearing aids on a headband within the first few months after birth. Surgery is not required for fitting a soft band device and can be performed in a single day in qualified centers. The sound from a headband bone conduction hearing device is not as good as the implanted variety, but it is close enough to normal sound to allow stimulation of the auditory system and speech development. The surface BCHA can be worn until the best CAAM treatment is determined two or three years in the future. Without using this device early and frequently, severe language and word formation effects will occur.

Many patients use a headband BCHA for their first three years before a surgically created ear canal is performed. This approach maximizes the first three years of speech development.

Some parents choose to use a headband BCHA in single-sided CAAM as well. Undoubtedly, the sound from the surface device stimulates the CAAM inner ear and brain pathway. While we believe this will be proven beneficial, not enough data exists at this time to recommend this strategy for all patients. We do know, however, that a headband BCHA must be introduced early (preferably under six to eight months of age) or a child will not accept it. Two- or three-year-olds simply remove the device every time a parent tries to put it on! Conversely, if children use devices from a young age, they accept them as part of their normal lives.

Microtia Repair Options

Two main methods of surgical outer ear reconstruction exist today and are detailed below – rib graft repair and PPE repair. Your choice of technique to reconstruct the outer ear malformation affects the timing of atresia repair if your child is a candidate for an ear canal surgery. Ear canal surgery follows rib graft repair. Ear canal surgery occurs before or at the same time as PPE repair. Consultation with a plastic surgeon adept in the technique is an important and necessary part of treatment planning. Your decision should be made by the time the CT scan is read at 2.5 years of age.

Plastic surgeons usually perform only one technique and can feel rather strongly about which method is best. Expect to receive conflicting information if you talk to different plastic surgeons, especially if they use different techniques. I have tried to give you some advantages and disadvantages of the different techniques below and to help you know what to ask of your chosen plastic surgeon/s. We remain available to help you sort through different recommendations from different surgeons should you become frustrated or confused.

I advise you to ask how many surgical repairs a plastic surgeon has performed when you have a consultation. It takes quite a number of cases to become good at microtia repair. You should seek to avoid a disastrous result from inexperienced surgeons operating on your child with good intentions.

Be aware that a high percentage of plastic surgeons know little about hearing or the importance of early hearing restoration for speech and language and brain development. (That's understandable since hearing loss is not a topic of education in plastic surgery training programs.) Consequently, your plastic surgeon may not factor in this aspect of your child's function and future when recommending treatment. Some plastic surgeons have educated themselves about the effect of hearing impairment on their patients and do a good job considering it in treatment planning. In my experience, it is best to consult your otologist regarding any advice given by a plastic surgeon about hearing.

The malformed portion of the outer ear is sometimes called the pinna. Three options for reconstructions exist:

- External prosthesis
- Rib graft implant
- Porous Polyethylene Implant (PPE) (MEDPOR™, Supor™)

Differences between techniques are outlined briefly below. You must select a method of outer ear reconstruction before you can make the final plan for hearing.

Comparison of Outer Ear Reconstruction Options

	When outer ear procedure begins	Number of surgeries required	Kind of surgeon needed for outer ear procedure	When ear canal surgery can occur
External prosthesis	Any age	None	Prosthetics specialists	Before or after fitting. An external prosthesis can be made to fit around the ear canal.
Rib graft implant	Five or six years	Three to four	Plastic surgeon	After (upon completion of outer the series of three to four ear surgeries)
PPE implant	Three years	One	Plastic surgeon	Before or at the same time

Worldwide, more patients receive rib graft implantation than other techniques. Rib graft repair has been around since the 1960s, and more surgeons are familiar with it. Over the past decade, however, there has been a shift away from the traditional method of microtia repair in centers of excellence like ours. More parents select PPE implantation than rib graft implantation in our patients. Few patients use an external prosthesis unless they aren't candidates for surgical reconstruction. Examples where prostheses are a good option include missing ears, burned ears, or in ears that lack the tissues necessary for successful reconstruction (as determined by a plastic surgeon).

Almost always, different surgeons are required to perform atresia repair and microtia repair on each patient. For best results, seamless coordination and communication are needed between these teams. Without it, one surgeon can make another surgeon's job difficult or impossible. For example, if jaw surgery is done before microtia surgery and the artery needed for outer ear reconstruction is damaged, PPE implantation can be difficult or impossible, and a different technique may have to be used.

I work with surgeons who use each technique. Frequently, parents ask my objective opinion of the three techniques. By describing each, and listing the major advantages and disadvantages of each, I hope to give you some assistance in selecting your own best choice.

External Prosthesis

What Is It?

An outer ear model can be made of rubbery plastic. It is extremely realistic and can match an existing ear nearly identically. To get a sense for the technology, imagine a Hollywood movie where costumes and amazing effects are created.

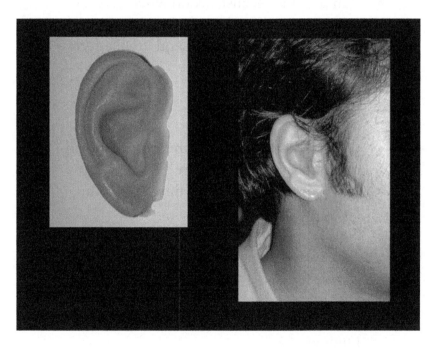

An example of an outer ear prosthesis, held in position by glues.

How Is It Used?

Users wear the prosthesis each day and remove it each night. The device remains in place over the existing microtia ear or around a created ear canal. Two methods are used to secure the prosthesis. Glues are the most common method. Alternatively, magnets can be used to hold the external prosthesis in the correct location. The magnets require a surgical procedure to place them. After healing, the external prosthesis is created with corresponding magnets to hold it in position.

Advantages

- Can provide reconstruction when surgical options are not possible
- Provide the most realistic and lifelike reconstruction

Disadvantages

- Can fall off during wear and expose the underlying ear malformation
- Daily applications can be time consuming and difficult
- Natural skin tones change with the hot and cold seasons, so at least two different suntan shades are usually needed.
- Due to wear, damage, or loss, multiple prostheses will be necessary during a patient's lifetime

Rib Graft

In rib graft surgery, a portion of a rib is removed from the chest wall to construct an ear form. This form is then implanted under the existing skin of the microtia ear after removal of the malformed cartilage tissue. One or two ears

can be constructed using the rib graft technique. A sufficient rib from one side of the anterior chest is used for each
ear.

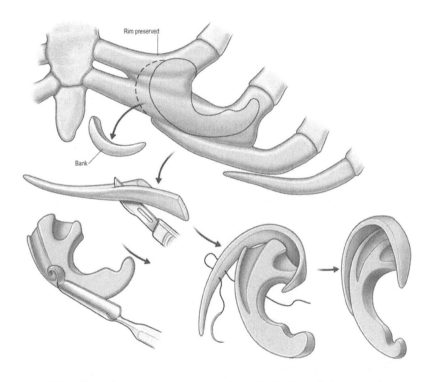

For rib graft outer ear reconstruction, rib cartilage is harvested
from the anterior chest wall and used to create a custom scaffold for
implantation under the skin.

Children must be at least five or six years of age, or
even older if they have small bodies, for enough cartilage
to be present to construct an ear. Three or four stages of
reconstruction are performed, each with its own surgery.

1. The first is the removal of the rib and the
    creation and implantation of the ear form.

2. The ear lobe (which is usually relatively normal but in the wrong position in a microtia ear) is moved to the correct position after the cartilage implant heals.
3. The ear is lifted with a skin graft behind the cartilage to help the ear project away from the head and match the opposite side.
4. Some surgeons add a fourth reconstruction to add a tragus, which is a small piece of cartilage normally located in front of the ear canal. Some surgeons perform this step during the third surgery.

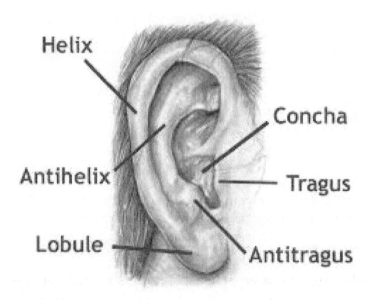

A diagram of the normal anatomical landmarks of the outer ear.

Ear canal reconstruction must take place after rib graft surgery for the rib graft technique to heal appropriately. (See Atresia Repair Surgery below.)

Each stage requires healing before the next surgery can be performed. On average, Global Hearing's patients who select rib graft surgery average 3.6 surgeries before an ear canal is created. Our average age for ear canal creation with ear rib graft microtia repair is 11.6 years.

As you know from the critical period of development section above, 11.6 years is beyond the period of normal development of important portions of hearing, such as speech and language. If rib graft microtia repair is selected, it is important to stimulate the ear being reconstructed with a bone conduction hearing device (a description of this technology is below) until the ear canal is reconstructed.

Advantages

- Since rib is our own tissue, reaction to the material is minimal. This technique avoids the use of foreign material in the body. The new ear is effectively a transplant of the patient's own tissue, and there is little risk the body will not accept it or heal well.
- The rate of implant exposure — in other words, when the implant protrudes through the skin and makes another surgery for removal and replacement necessary — is 1% for patients.
- More resistant to traumatic injury than PPE. Both techniques can suffer injury, which may require revision surgery.
- Rib graft surgery does not limit the activities of a patient.

- The reconstructed ear has a better sensation on the ear and surrounding skin. Because rib graft does not require the dissection of tissue from under the scalp, the risk of hair loss or scalp thinning is not present.
- It is rare to have to replace a rib graft implant.
- Infection around surgery is less than 1% of cases.

Disadvantages

- Due to the extended schedule of rib graft surgery, outer ear reconstruction is not accomplished until after the age that other children often tease others for how they look physically.
- Multiple surgical procedures are difficult and can be psychologically challenging for children through early teenage years.
- Scarring and pain are an impact of harvesting cartilage from the chest wall.
- Since rib graft microtia surgery must be completed before ear canal surgery, hearing is not restored until after ten years of age, when the critical period of hearing and speech development has passed. We have seen a difference, particularly in hearing in noise, in patients who have had hearing restored later. These patients are left with permanent hearing and functional deficits. It is possible to minimize, but not alleviate,

such effects by using a bone conduction hearing aid until the hearing is restored.

- Compared to PPE, a rib graft has a less normal appearance. This is mainly because the ears made with rib graft are usually situated against the head and do not project like a normal ear. From the side, they can be natural. From the front or from any other angle, it is clearly abnormal.

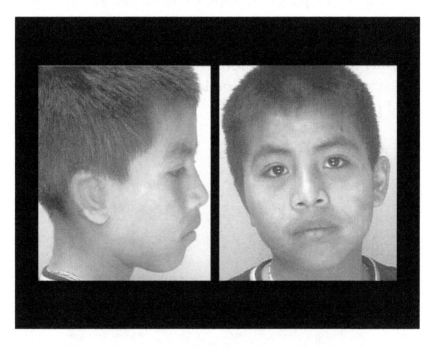

An example of a patient with unilateral right CAAM after outer ear reconstruction with rib graft. Note the lack of natural projection away from the head, compared to the normal left ear.

- The rate of narrowing of the ear canal after ear canal surgery (called stenosis and described below in the section on ear canal re-

pair) is higher with rib graft versus PPE implantation.
- Rib may resorb over time, causing the implant to decrease in size or to deform

Porous Polyethylene Implantation (PPE)

Surgical reconstruction is accomplished with a man-made
material designed for implantation. The material is constructed with a porous design, so blood vessels and tissue
grow into it as it heals. The material is made by at least two
companies and comes in two pieces. The pieces are welded
together in the operating room to create an ear of the shape
and size desired. The PPE implant is then placed in the desired position.

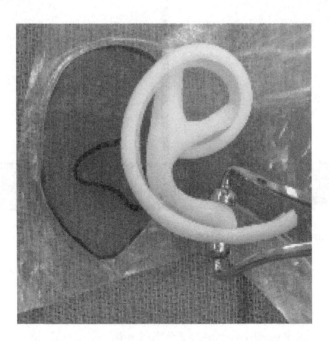

*PPE ear implant under construction sized to a template drawn to
match the normal opposite ear.*

A tissue membrane normally situated between the skin of the scalp and the bone of the skull is dissected free during surgery and left attached to its blood supply just above the normal ear. The membrane is placed over the PPE implant, and a suction is used to shrink wrap the membrane onto the PPE implant. Skin grafts are taken from other body portions and sewn together over the membrane flap. Then they are also suctioned onto the membrane flap's surface to cover the PPE implant. The membrane flap's blood supply provides oxygen to the skin grafts until after they heal, as the arrangement creates a lining of living tissue.

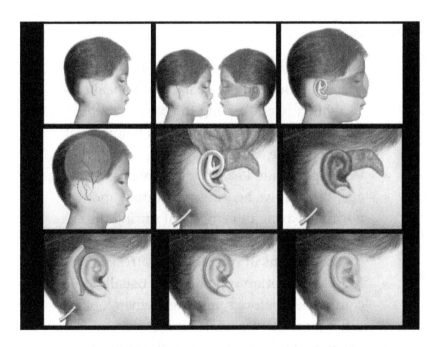

The overall steps of PPE microtia repair. First, a template is made (if applicable) from the opposite ear, which is used to customize the PPE implant. A tissue flap is dissected and brought down to cover the implant, holding it in place. Finally, skin grafts are used to cover the newly constructed ear.

Ear canal surgery can be performed before PPE reconstruction or at the same time. (See Atresia Repair and Combined Atresia Microtia Repair sections below, respectively.) Ear canal healing should be allowed for a minimum of four months (six months of separation is ideal) before undergoing PPE reconstruction if your treatment plan includes separate surgeries. Ear canal reconstruction after PPE puts the PPE implant at higher risk. While we have performed canal surgery after PPE implantations in a few select patients, we recommend against this approach due to increased risk of complication to the PPE implant.

Advantages

- Since PPE implantation does not rely on the tissue surrounding the ear canal to heal correctly before addressing the ear canal, the canal surgery can be performed before or at the same time as PPE.
- When performed as early as three years of age, PPE allows hearing restoration and normal hearing development during the critical period, while also addressing the aesthetic concerns of microtia and atresia.
- PPE implantation can be and is usually accomplished before school age, when looking different from classmates is an issue.
- On average, 2.6 fewer surgical procedures are required for PPE than for rib graft implantation. This is less challenging psychologically and physically for children, for obvious reasons.

- The best PPE implant results are superior to rib graft implant results in mimicking normal ears. Mainly, this is due to how the reconstructed ears project from the skull to match the other ear from any angle.

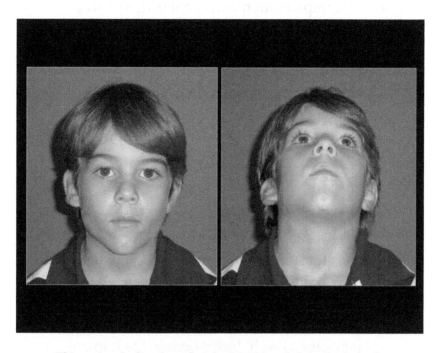

This patient had unilateral right CAAM and elected to have the outer ear reconstructed via PPE implantation. Notice the excellent symmetry of the ears, especially with regard to projection of the ear from the head. (Compare to the previous rib graft image.)

- PPE implantation is more easily coupled with an ear canal. Some rib graft implants can be incorrectly placed over the area where the ear canal ought to be. Since the ear canal should always be created either before or at the same time as PPE, we do not see the PPE being placed incorrectly over the ear canal.

- The rate of narrowing of the ear canal is lower with PPE implantation compared to rib graft implantation.
- PPE implantation and canal surgery can be performed in a single outpatient procedure, minimizing the number of surgeries without compromising excellent outcomes. We are currently the only team worldwide doing combined atresia and microtia repair in a single procedure (the CAM procedure).

Disadvantages

- PPE is as good a material as we currently have for implant construction. Nonetheless, it is still a foreign material, and problems can occur. The implant comes through the skin in 4% of patients. Usually, this occurs in the early postoperative period but may happen later as well. If this occurs, the implant can be covered with a small surgery that repositions local tissue. Rarely, a more significant surgery is needed to remove the implant and allow the skin to heal. In this case, the implant then needs to be replaced with a later surgery.
- The PPE is more apt to break with a blow to the ear. The framework that is surgically welded in the operating room can separate, causing a loss of form and/or a problem with

the tissue over the PPE implant. This is rare but may lead to a revision surgery with implant replacement.

- Infection rates around surgery are higher with PPE than rib graft. However, this infection rate is still low, involving less than 1% of cases.

The cosmetic appearance following microtia reconstruction is important to your choice. It can avoid significant psychological and social consequences for your child. However, experience has also taught me that, the older your child becomes, the more important their hearing function will be—both to them and to you. It's up to you to consider hearing, development, and future function in your decision-making process.

Direct Advice

I want to be sure you understand a mistake I see some families make. If parents focus only on the way an ear looks and do not address hearing early in the child's life, they almost always regret the effect on hearing later. I can promise you, having only one single hearing ear will impose limits on what your child can and should be in the future. The best strategy is to marry form AND function with the plan you are putting together.

Hearing Results Following Surgery

Expected hearing outcomes can be understood by correlating the chance of success based with a CT scan score. In

children who have a CT score of 5 or better, a high percentage (>95%) of children have improved hearing. The
hearing can be partial or can even return the hearing to the
normal range. It is important to understand that even the
best results of atresia repair surgery do not return the hearing to the level of a normal ear, but it can come close. Following surgery, the brain uses the data from the 'new' ear
and integrates it with the normal signal coming from the
unaffected ear in cases of unilateral CAAM. In cases of bilateral CAAM, the hearing levels frequently allow children
to stop using devices such as the soft band BAHA or
Ponto, permitting them to live device-free.

Analysis of our surgical cases has produced the following data. Patients who have a CT scan score of 8–10 have
the highest chance (80%) of reaching the normal range of
hearing, which is defined as 0–30 dB on the audiogram. In
other words, 8 out of 10 patients with scores in this range
will achieve hearing in the normal range. The remaining 2
out of 10 patients have high odds of hearing being
improved but hear outside the normal range in that ear.
Patients with a score of 6 or 7 also have a good chance
(67%) of reaching the 0-30 dB goal for hearing. Again, note
that some patients who do not reach the 0-30 dB range can
frequently have a middle ear bone repair performed as a
second surgery to elevate the hearing to normal ranges. In
our patients, a second surgery has been necessary in 6% (or
1 in 17) of cases. If the hearing does not reach 0-30 dB, other methods of supplying hearing to the ear are available to
us, including use of air conduction hearing devices as discussed previously in this book.

Children with a score of 5 have just under a 50%
chance of reaching desired levels. Scores of 4 or less rarely

allow significant improvement in hearing. This is the reason we do not recommend surgery with CT scores of 4 or less.

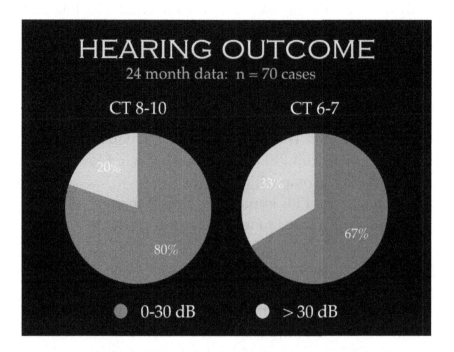

HEARING OUTCOME
24 month data: n = 70 cases

CT 8-10   CT 6-7

20%   33%

80%   67%

● 0-30 dB   ● > 30 dB

Hearing outcome based on CT scan J-score. The dark blue percentages shown are the fraction of patients in each category who achieved hearing in the normal range of 0-30 dB after canal surgery. The light blue percentages represent patients whose hearing was outside the 0-30 dB range. Still, almost all patients have improved hearing overall after canal surgery.

Future Considerations

I believe the future is bright for a revolution in microtia repair. New biomaterial techniques use the patient's own tissue to create an ear that is more realistic in texture and shape. For example, some companies are working on material that is 3D printed. In this way, an ear can be hyper-customized. Say, for example, your child has single-sided CAAM. Their reconstructed ear can be matched nearly exactly to the existing ear. Or, if your child has bilateral CAAM, perhaps their ears can be the same shape as yours!

Currently, both rib graft implants and PPE implants are stiff and do not bend. If a material can be made of the patient's own tissue and can be made more flexible, the ear may look more natural and, importantly, may be more resistant to trauma. This strategy will also reduce the exposure rates seen with PPE, as the material is not foreign and will be more biocompatible.

I predict the PPE implant surgical technique will continue and will be used to implant newer, better biomaterial outer ears in the next 3–10 years. While that is exciting, it creates other issues. For example, how long would you want to see data from patients with these newer implants before we can assume the technique holds up over time? What sort of late complications are there, AND how does it look after 10, 20, or even 30 years? At this time, we have more than 50 years of history with rib graft implants and more than 20 years of history with PPE implants. Still, it is exciting to see a new and better way on the horizon.

One common question is, "Can we reconstruct our child's ear canal and wait for outer ear technology to improve, and if so, how long should we wait?" Yes, if an ear canal is created, the outer ear reconstruction can wait for years. Some patients are currently choosing to have an ear canal only made in small children to enjoy the benefits of auditory and brain development during the critical period. They plan to observe the rapidly evolving technology of outer ear reconstruction before having surgery for the microtia component of CAAM.

Also, we have an adequate amount of experience now to know replacement of PPE implants is not a terribly difficult operation. When a PPE implant breaks, it is replaced by making a vertical incision and opening the skin pouch around it like a clam shell. The new implant is then inserted and the skin is closed. The incision heals quickly and beautifully in almost all instances. I see no reason an existing PPE implant could not be removed and replaced by new material of the exact same size in the future, should one become available.

Another potential combination of techniques may prove to be rib graft implantation following primary ear canal surgery, when canal surgery is performed first using a minimally invasive approach known as micro-incision canalplasty. This technique minimizes scarring around the site of the surgically created canal. Since the skin around the ear canal is not disturbed, this technique may permit placement of a rib graft in a second surgery later, allowing canal reconstruction to occur prior to rib graft surgery.

Treatment Decision Algorithm

This algorithm has proven helpful to parents in understanding their decisions regarding CAAM treatment. As you have now read about much of the information included in the algorithm, it should make sense. Note some small deviations in the algorithm's order are needed for some patients, and a personalized plan is always recommended. If you understand this, you are well on your way to understanding treatment decisions and choices for CAAM!

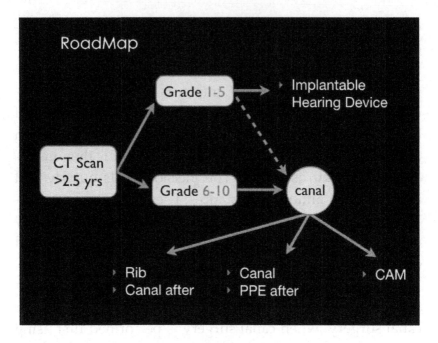

A road map to treatment plan options based on CT scan score.

Special Conditions Some CAAM Patients Have

Partial Ear Canal

Development of the ear canal begins within the first few weeks after conception. It's possible for the process to stop before it is fully complete. Most often, complete atresia (absence of the ear canal altogether) is the most common abnormality. In a small percentage of cases, however, the partial completion of development results in a partial formation of the ear canal.

Partial ear canals may be a short canal that is visible from the exterior but does not fully extend to an eardrum or may be partially present deep within the skull base without a connecting opening to the exterior. There may even be a partial eardrum present. In general, these patients can get some of the best hearing outcomes from surgery. However, the surgical procedure is harder than a complete atresia. Surgeons have to work around the present skin and other tissues that must be preserved. CT scans are necessary to evaluate partial canal development and for planning appropriate treatment. It is important to note that cholesteatomas occur at a higher rate in partial canal development than in complete atresia patients.

Cholesteatoma

As the ear canal and outer ear form in utero, the process can malfunction and produce a cyst of buried skin called a cholesteatoma. The trapped tissue forms a tumor either in the soft tissue around the malformed ear or deeper in the skull bone. The tumor is not cancerous but can cause significant damage if not removed. Over time, cholesteatomas grow and cause bone erosion around them. With enlargement, these destructive lesions can erode into the ear structures, such as the middle ear bones and facial nerve. Possible effects include facial paralysis, loss of hearing function in the involved ear, or severe balance disturbance. In advanced cases, the enlarging mass may erode into the brain cavity and threaten life. In some patients, cholesteatomas become infected and damage surrounding structures. Fortunately, this condition only occurs in a small percentage of cases. We must, however, rule out the presence of a cholesteatoma or patients who are at high risk for developing one in all cases as part of our evaluation.

Not all cholesteatomas can be diagnosed by examining the external microtia ear malformation. In some cases, a cholesteatoma can be present with no external signs whatsoever. It is also important to note that in some patients, a cholesteatoma can go undetected (until a complication occurs) if outer ear surgery is performed without first evaluating a CT scan for the presence of a tumor. Because of this, a CT scan is an essential part of evaluating patients with atresia and microtia.

For this reason, all CAAM patients should have a CT scan before any microtia or atresia repair surgeries are done.

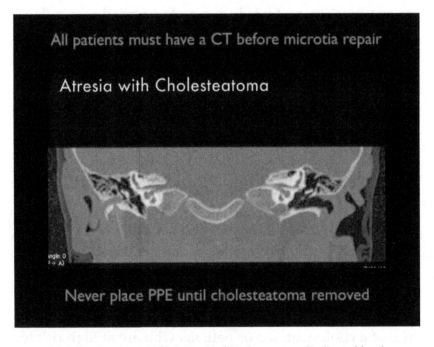

CT scan of patient with right-sided cholesteatoma (indicated by the red arrow). If present, cholesteatomas must be removed before any type of ear surgery is performed!

In some cases of small ear canals, creation of an outer ear can increase the chance a cholesteatoma will develop from a partially formed ear canal. An experienced otologist needs to make that decision, not a plastic surgeon. In other cases of small ear canals, an outer ear can be created with a low risk of cholesteatoma induction.

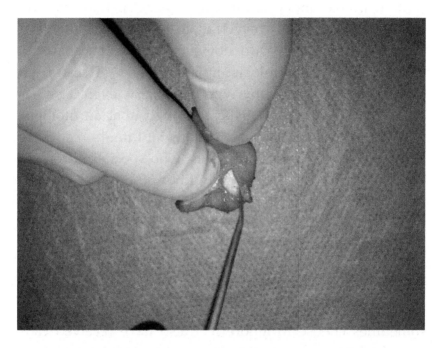

A cholesteatoma after removal in the operating room. Note the visible skin lining of the tumor.

Please insist on a CT for your child! Some of the world's most experienced outer ear reconstructive surgeons regularly violate this rule and perform outer ear reconstruction without checking for these rare tumors first. Even the surgeons I work most closely with have made this mistake. Again, if you are told that a visual examination alone is sufficient to make sure a cholesteatoma is not present, you are dealing with a surgeon who is not fully aware of these tumors and their consequences.

Each year, I am referred patients who have never had a CT scan, yet had growing cholesteatomas that caused severe complications. In addition to being a threat to function and life, the presence of an undiscovered cholesteatoma under a microtia reconstruction (via rib graft or PPE implant) may lead to loss of the outer ear. Since plastic surgeons do not ever read CT scans with CAAM, a qualified otologist must review a CT scan from every patient prior to any type of surgery, even if an ear canal is not planned. I suggest strongly that an otologist who knows to look for these congenital tumors read your child's CT scan. Even radiologists, who specialize in reading X-rays and CT scans, rarely know these tumors exist and frequently miss them when reviewing scans of patients with CAAM.

Cholesteatomas are easily missed at the time of outer ear reconstruction. I have dealt with this complication from some of the world's best plastic surgeons who specialize in CAAM who either don't understand the entity or sometimes choose to ignore it. I also have received calls directly from the operating rooms of multiple other surgeons who have discovered this unsuspected tumor while in surgery and don't know how to deal with it. If an unsuspected tumor is found during microtia repair, the surgery should be stopped and an experienced otologist enlisted to remove the cholesteatoma before proceeding. Since an experienced otologist is usually not available at a moment's notice to go to the OR, a separate later surgery to remove the cholesteatoma is generally required, followed by a third surgery to complete the first stage of microtia repair.

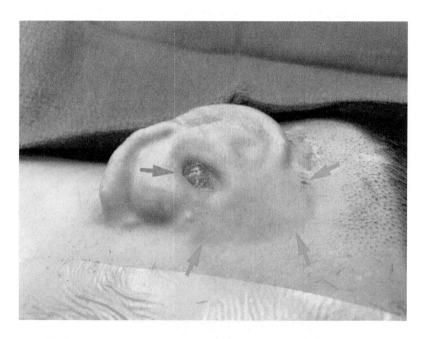

PPE reconstruction was placed over a known cholesteatoma by a surgeon and family who ignored recommendations for cholesteatoma removal. Three years later, the tumor grew under the implant, threatening the child's life and requiring PPE implant removal.

Cholesteatomas must be removed completely to ensure a child's safety. Even one cell of tissue left in the tissue or bone of the skull base will grow back and reform a tumor. Otologists use operating microscopes for ear microsurgery to remove cholesteatomas. The tumor frequently extends deep into the bone or neck structures where outer ear surgeons do not operate regularly. Because of this, they should never be removed without an otologist familiar with these structures, and only under an operating microscope. Plastic surgeons do not use microscopes for microtia repair and are unfamiliar with microsurgical techniques. They should not attempt cholesteatoma removal. As with many surgical procedures, the best chance of successfully and permanently addressing this threatening condition is to do the first surgery correctly.

In cases where an ear canal is not possible or is not selected, a cholesteatoma MUST be removed before microtia reconstruction is performed. Cholesteatoma is one of the few CAAM situations that can threaten the life of your child. The condition must be diagnosed before undertaking surgery of any kind.

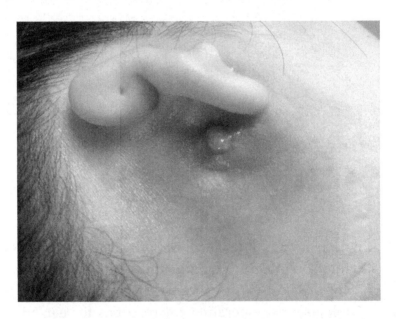

Canal cholesteatoma that has become infected and has broken through the skin over the mastoid bone. Surgery and antibiotics were required to remove the cholesteatoma and stop the infection.

Fibrous Incudo-Stapedial (IS) Joint

Around 2005, I began using a new technology to look into patients' middle ears while in the operating room. We always use a powerful surgical microscope for all operations for CAAM. This technology, however—a tiny camera and recording equipment—allowed me to see things I could not see otherwise.

> *We found something interesting that surgeons had not known for years: the joint between the second and third middle ear bones was formed incorrectly in a significant number of cases (26.7%).*

This was the first time this malformation was noted in CAAM patients and published—a situation that may have been responsible for the poor and unexplained hearing results we found in some patients. The medical paper we produced with the help of one of our excellent fellow physicians describing this finding was published in 2014.[11]

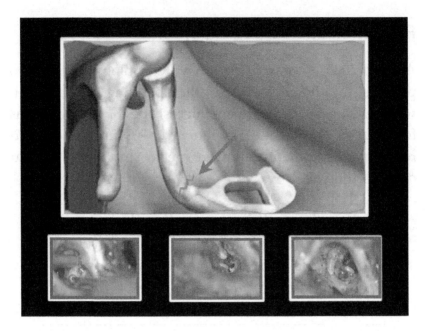

Middle ear bones with commonly affected area of fibrous union.

Can We Improve the Condition?

We set out to determine if we could improve surgical results in this condition. This was a significant step forward in understanding this abnormality present in the middle ear bones of a substantial number of patients. We were the first to discover this issue and, as a result of our findings, made significant progress in finding a cause of poor hearing outcomes in 27% of our patients! For years, surgeons had not known about this anatomic abnormality and, as a result, could not correctly identify the cause of less than optimal hearing outcomes in patients affected by this condition. It turns out the condition was a major cause in many cases when CAAM patients' hearing did not improve adequately despite successful surgery.

Below, you see the images from one of the surgeries where we found this abnormality.

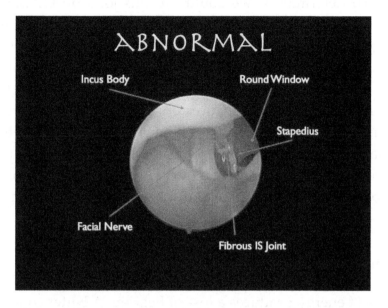

Abnormal fibrous incudo-stapedial (IS) joint under the microscope.

Normally, the joint between the incus (the second middle ear bone) and the stapes (the third middle ear bone) measures less than 1 mm and is the smallest joint in the body. Because the joint involves bone touching bone with the smallest joint in the body in between, any sound vibration from the eardrum travels to the first middle ear bone (called the malleus), and then to the incus and stapes, and finally into the inner ear. In this example, the joint between the incus and the stapes is not bone on bone but, rather, is composed of a short length of scar tissue. Instead of the firm connection normally present, this tissue is flexible, and a significant portion of energy is lost in vibration. This means that sound waves conducted through the hearing chain are lost at this connection point, and hearing does not reach desired levels.

To determine if we could see this joint on CT scans prior to surgery, we went to our digital repository and reviewed hundreds of scans. We found that it was impossible to be 100% sure of the status of the IS joint based on a CT scan alone. While CT scans are the gold standard for evaluating the bony structures of the middle ear, the reality is that this joint is mere millimeters in size and is too small to identify for certain if the tissue is normal or not based on CT scan imaging alone. For that reason, we only know the status of the IS joint for sure when we see it in the operating room.

How Do We Fix It?

Loss of energy produces a loss of hearing. A better connection between the middle ear bones is needed to achieve optimal hearing. To treat this issue, I developed several titanium prostheses to allow us to "bridge the gap" and improve hearing results in patients with abnormal IS joints. Here you see some of the prostheses which measure only 1–3 mm in size. They are in use today for fibrous IS joint reconstruction. Since the middle ear bones are fully grown at birth, the prosthesis does not have to be replaced as the child grows. They last for life.

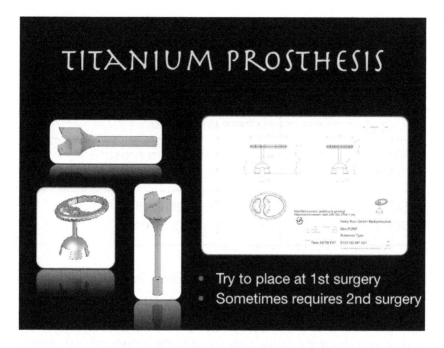

Various customized middle ear bone reconstruction prostheses.

To determine if we needed to repair all cases of fibrous IS joint, regardless of severity, we performed a study to assess IS joint status and hearing outcomes. This data would help us know when to use these new prostheses and when to leave the joint as is. We noticed some patients had good hearing tests despite having fibrous IS joint, while others did not have as good of hearing outcomes after surgery. Through advanced statistical analysis of our patients' reconstruction outcomes, we developed the following guidelines:

Normal IS Joint	No reconstruction
Mild Fibrous IS Joint	No reconstruction; wait for hearing test four to five months after surgery to determine if a second surgery is needed
Moderate Fibrous IS Joint	Reconstruct with a prosthesis during the first surgery
Severe Fibrous IS Joint	Reconstruct with a prosthesis during the first surgery

In patients who have a mild fibrous IS joint, a good percentage of patients will have adequate post-operative hearing. Other patients enjoy improved but not maximally improved hearing and require another surgery to repair the middle ear bones with the placement of a titanium prosthesis. This applies to 6% of Global Hearing patients. The revision surgery in these cases goes through the newly created ear canal, where the eardrum is lifted and the pros-thetic repair is performed. Healing is much more rapid than the first surgery. The research to determine when to replace the joint at the time of the first surgery saves many patients the necessity of having a second surgery.

Hearing results with the prostheses can be great and rival those of normal middle ear bones. In fact, some of our best hearing results are seen with middle ear bone recon-struction. Middle ear bone implants are designed to last a lifetime but, on occasion, can become displaced, requiring revision surgery to replace them and restore previous hearing levels.

A Summary of Fibrous IS Joint Abnormality

Here is a summary of what we know about the fibrous IS joint abnormality:

Fibrous IS joint abnormalities can be a source of hearing impairment in a significant percentage of patients, even with successful ear canal and eardrum surgeries, and can be easily missed.

Reconstruction and better hearing can be achieved with custom-designed titanium middle ear implants.

CT scans before surgery occasionally can reveal the status of the IS joint. Usually, however, the small area can only be seen with 100% certainty in the operating room with special equipment.

Moderate and severe fibrous IS joint abnormalities are repaired at the first surgery because significant hearing loss will remain present if the problem is not addressed.

In a small percentage of mild fibrous IS joint surgeries, a second surgery will be needed to achieve maximum hearing results. However, most of these cases will achieve adequate hearing with the first surgery and do not require an additional procedure.

Hemi-Facial Microsomia (HFM) & Facial Asymmetry

In many patients, the side of the facial structures affected by CAAM will be less developed than the opposite normal side. In bilateral CAAM, both sides of the face may be un-derdeveloped. The structures affected are the soft tissue of the cheek and face, the jaw, and the midface bone structure called the maxilla.

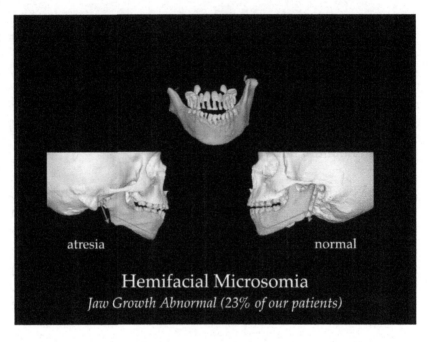

atresia   normal

Hemifacial Microsomia
Jaw Growth Abnormal (23% of our patients)

Hemifacial Microsomia, or asymmetry of the bone and soft tissue structures of the face, is sometimes associated with CAAM.

In most situations, the difference from the normal side is slight. In severe situations, there can be a marked un-derdevelopment of the affected side. The "M" and the sec-ond "A" of the HEAR MAPS grading system indicates how severe the abnormality is.

23% of individuals evaluated by our team for CAAM have a facial asymmetry. Not all of them require treatment.

Severe asymmetry may be classified as Hemi-Facial Microsomia (HFM). Also, one particular syndrome—Goldenhar Syndrome—can present as HFM but also may involve malformations of the kidney, thyroid, lungs, and, occasionally, the spine. Neither HFM nor Goldenhar Syndrome is associated with intellectual disability. Genetic testing is available for Goldenhar Syndrome.

The jaw, midface, and facial soft tissue develop over the first 10–12 years of life, the majority of which occurs during the first 6 years. In patients born with mild asymmetry, the amount of asymmetry can become either more normal or less normal over the first few years of life. Patients born with no asymmetry rarely develop significant asymmetry and never develop severe asymmetry or jaw problems. In other words, children are born with the abnormality or not, and, in some cases, it can get worse with childhood growth. In others, it may improve with time.

Those with severe asymmetry, especially underdevelopment of the mandible, may have compromise of the space in the throat where air passes to the lungs during sleep. Any snoring in a child is abnormal, and a test can be done to determine if these patients suffer from obstructive sleep apnea due to a small airway. The test is called a sleep study (or polysomnogram) and is done overnight. Monitors observe a child's air passage during sleep.

Surgical procedures can alter the jaw bone and face to correct abnormalities to normal, or near-normal, function and appearance. Craniofacial surgeons perform these procedures.

A member of Global Hearing's team invented a device that lengthens jaws in certain patients.

Usually, surgery for HFM is delayed until the teenage years, but severe cases may require early surgery. Consultation with a craniofacial surgeon may be indicated if a moderate or severe asymmetry exists. Should you be evaluated by our team, we will advise you on the best course of action. Early surgery *must* be coordinated with ear surgery, so the tissues and blood vessels needed for the canal and ear reconstructions are not damaged.

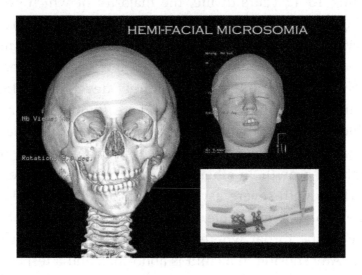

CT and reconstructed image with soft tissue showing underdevelopment of the jaw and soft tissues in Hemi-Facial Microsomia. The device at bottom-right is temporarily surgically implanted to lengthen the jaw.

In patients with mild asymmetry, where the jaw bone structure and face do not need to change, a simple procedure can make the face appear more even. Via liposuction, fat can be removed from the abdomen through a small incision in the umbilicus or belly button. This fat is then injected into the soft tissue of the underdeveloped side of the face. Fat grafting can be done more than once if needed. In some cases, surgery to lengthen the bones of the jaw/face can be performed in combination with fat grafting.

Ear Infections

Middle ear infections are known medically as Otitis Media (OM). In this condition, fluid fills the middle ear, often after a cold or viral infection. The fluid becomes infected, and white blood cells come into the fluid to fight the infection. In normal ears, this increase in fluid volume generates pressure in the middle ear and presses on the eardrum, which hurts quite a lot. Most parents have encountered pediatric ear infections, as they are common.

When present, the infection and fluid cause a temporary decrease in hearing by affecting the eardrum, which doesn't move as well as usual in response to sound. Usually, the fluid begins to clear within a few days after starting antibiotics, and hearing improves. In some cases, fluid remains in the ear and hearing stays low.

Just about every child gets OM at some point. You can reduce its incidence by keeping up with pediatric immunizations, avoiding smoking around the child, and reducing colds (which is a tough thing). We want to treat any ear infections promptly to return the hearing to normal as soon as possible in a normal ear.

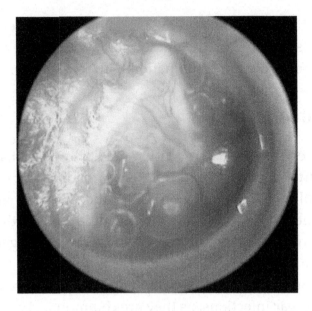

Mild ear infection with fluid and bubbles in the middle ear behind the eardrum.

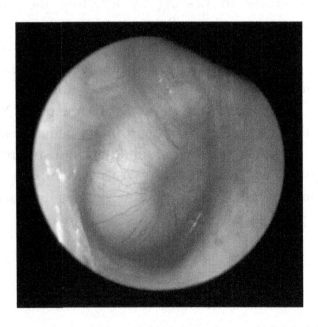

Acute ear infection with pus behind the eardrum, which is bulging outward.

In ears where the fluid stays more than two months, or if infections appear more than three times in one year, we recommend placement of a Tympanostomy Tube (also called a "grommet" or "pressure equalizing tube"). It promotes the removal and healing of any fluid in the middle ear and can markedly reduce the chance of future ear infections. The downside of this surgical procedure is small. Only 1% of patients will have a hole remaining in their eardrum after the tube naturally falls out six to nine months later. In the case of a remaining hole, it can easily be fixed.

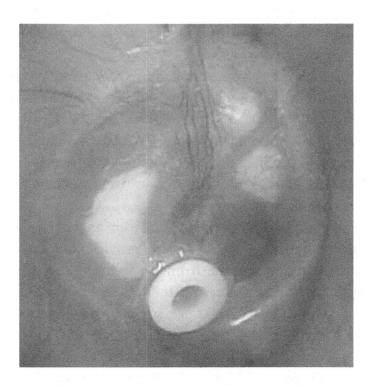

Ear with tympanostomy tube in place. The white cloudy areas are scarring present in the eardrum, left over from prior infections. These scars do not typically harm hearing.

Tympanostomy tube placement is the most common procedure in children in the United States and can be performed by virtually any ear, nose, and throat (ENT) doctor or pediatric ENT doctor (also called otorhinolaryngologists). The procedure takes less than 10 minutes to complete under mild anesthesia so that the child will be still and the doctor can work on the ear safely.

Children with recurring OM should be evaluated for enlargement of the tonsils and/or adenoids. These structures can harbor chronic infections or, if enlarged sufficiently, can obstruct the opening of the eustachian tubes. The eustachian tubes bring air to the middle ear. If you've ever held your nose and popped your ear, you've interacted with the eustachian tube.

Obstruction of the eustachian tube can produce chronic fluid and/or infections of the middle ear. If these structures are abnormal, surgical removal of the tonsils and adenoids is a good idea before CAAM canal surgery. If they grow to problematic sizes after CAAM, which is unusual, they can be removed then as well—usually by an ENT doctor close to your home.

You may be wondering if OM can affect the CAAM ear (or ears). Yes, it can. A health provider can look in a normal ear and see the eardrum. By seeing fluid behind an eardrum and/or infection and redness, we can make a diagnosis of OM. In a CAAM ear, we have no ear canal, nor do we have an eardrum to examine. While a CT can show the presence of fluid in the middle ear, we don't do CT scans to diagnose OM in CAAM ears. If your child has CAAM and is sick with a fever and your pediatrician cannot find any other source to explain the fever, assume OM is present and treat with oral antibiotics.

Each month, we get emails stating a patient has developed an infection in a reconstructed CAAM ear many months after surgery. Usually, this is an outer ear canal infection affecting the skin of the canal itself—called Otitis Externa (OE)—but it can be OM. The rate of occurrence of OM appears to be the same in reconstructed CAAM ears as it is in normal children and is treated the same. If an infection is present in a reconstructed CAAM ear, ask a local doctor to examine the ear to determine whether the canal (OE) or middle ear (OM) is affected. In OE, germs infect the skin placed in the ear canal, causing drainage from the ear canal. Almost always, this occurs when the ear has not been cleaned enough. If the natural debris produced by the skin graft builds up, germs can thrive. By removing the excess debris and applying antibiotic drops, the infection is almost always eliminated. In OM, oral antibiotics are indicated to treat the infection. Sometimes both oral antibiotics and antibiotic drops may be needed.

Hearing Loss with Single-Sided CAAM

Your early hearing test or audiogram performed by an audiologist should test both ears. If the "good" ear in single-sided CAAM has a hearing loss (as it does in 23% of cases in our worldwide database), it is important to determine the cause, and fix it promptly, if possible.

Even a small hearing loss affects language development in the first three years of life, and potentially permanently. If your child has single-sided CAAM, she or he relies heavily on the normal ear to hear and develop language, until the CAAM ear is brought to functional hearing levels. If this additional hearing loss is present in the ear not affected with CAAM, we may need to add additional treatment to avoid a severe speech and language delay. Consultation with your team should focus on promptly getting the hearing in the "good" ear into the normal range, and on keeping it there as many days a year as possible.

Bilateral CAAM

Worldwide, 10% of patients have bilateral CAAM. These children require bone conduction hearing devices on a headband to hear as early as possible. Several types of these devices are available around the world. Not all of them are good quality nor do they all produce good hearing and speech development. Global Hearing fits such children within a few weeks of birth. By stimulating the inner ear in this way, speech can develop, and the brain begins development as well.

When CAAM is present in both ears, the HEAR MAPS evaluation score and treatment algorithm is determined for each ear individually. Usually, both ears have the same amount of development, CT scores, hearing test results, etc., but not always. As treatment plans are put together, special considerations are made to reduce the number of treatments.

Remember, *surface bone conduction devices (such as the soft band BAHA or Ponto devices) must be started early in life, or irreversible developmental abnormalities will result.*

Sleep Apnea

When a person's airway is too small, an inadequate amount of air passes into the lungs when they sleep. This can cause a dangerous condition that leads to poor growth and development and can affect ear function as well.

Any snoring in a child is abnormal and should be investigated. Children with CAAM are at higher risk of sleep apnea due to small jaws, enlarged tonsils, and enlarged adenoids. Correcting these abnormalities will help these children grow and function normally and will create better outcomes for ear surgery.

An otorhinolaryngologist (or ENT physician) can evaluate your child for sleep apnea. In many cases, an overnight sleep test is done in a center to study the air movement during sleep and to help evaluate for this condition. Note also that large tonsils and adenoids can cause recurrent ear infections and middle ear fluid, as well as sleep apnea.

Your local ENT surgeon may evaluate your child for treatment. First-level treatment includes removal of the tonsils and adenoids. Sometimes, a larger airway is needed, and a craniofacial surgeon may become involved if tonsil and adenoid removal do not solve the issue.

Facial Nerve Weakness

In rare situations, the facial nerve on the side of CAAM is weak, and facial expressions can be affected. Usually, this condition implies a more severe abnormality of inner ear structures, as the facial nerve runs through the inner and middle ear. Otologists are the medical professionals that treat facial nerve conditions.

A CT scan is still necessary for these patients, and some patients are nevertheless candidates for canal surgery. However, a weakness of the facial nerve makes it more likely a patient will have a low CT score and not be a candidate for a canal. Some patients with facial nerve weakness are good candidates to have an ear canal created, with excellent results. As you would expect, should canal surgery not be an option, other methods for getting hearing to an ear also remain possibilities. Usually, the facial nerve can be seen on a CT scan, and its position can be mapped. If the facial nerve is in the path where an ear canal would be created, it can be a reason not to do surgery. Careful attention is always paid to the facial nerve, but extra care must be used if the facial nerve is in a high-risk position.

Some surgical techniques can improve facial nerve function in some patients. Overall, most cases of facial nerve weakness are better left as they are at birth. In some situations, special care of the eye may be needed if the eyelid does not close well. Customized planning is needed by an otologist if this condition is present.

Mixed Hearing Loss/SNHL

In a small percentage of those born with CAAM, a "mixed hearing loss" is present. This term is used when the hearing loss is a mixture of two different types of hearing loss: a conductive loss caused by the absence of an ear canal, PLUS a sensorineural hearing loss caused by weakness of the hearing nerve. A hearing test will show the condition of the inner ear hearing nerve and is critical to evaluating the potential to hear with the creation of an ear canal. If the hearing nerve weakness is too great, an ear canal may not be worth pursuing. If the hearing nerve loss is mild or moderate, a canal and hearing aid after healing from surgery may be the only option for good hearing in the ear.

Chapter in Review

Begin treatment as soon as possible and select the best possible team.

Remain calm and confident when communicating with your child about surgery. Offer age-appropriate details, just not too many.

A variety of devices and microtia repair options are available. As available treatments continue to improve, it is important that your treatment plan leaves available to you as many future options as possible.

Be sure to have your child evaluated for other conditions associated with CAAM, such as cholesteatoma. Many doctors do not know to look for such a condition. Missing their presence can ultimately cause significant harm to your child.

Chapter 5

Bringing It All Together

Chapter At-A-Glance

BEST PRACTICES: Benchmarks for the best treatment available

OTHER RESOURCES: International conference and remote/in-house consultations

What's the Best Treatment?

The chart below ranks treatment options by their proximity to "normal" hearing, with #1 being best/closest:

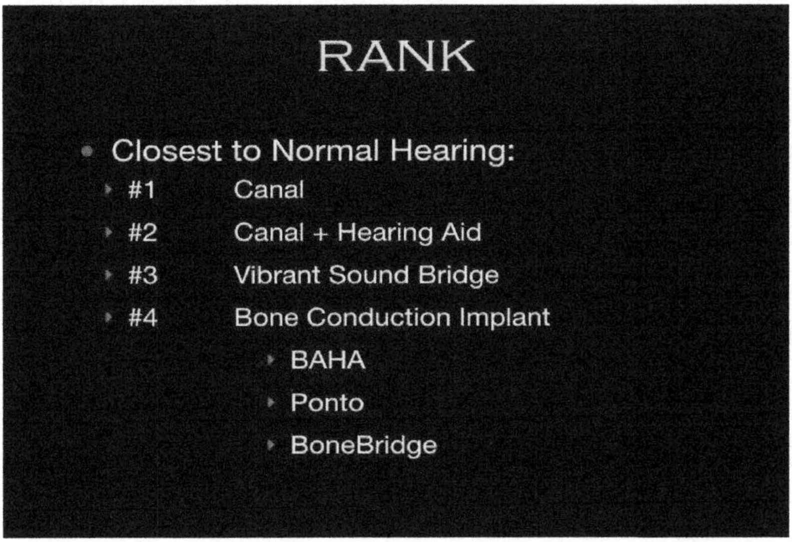

RANK

- **Closest to Normal Hearing:**
  - #1   Canal
  - #2   Canal + Hearing Aid
  - #3   Vibrant Sound Bridge
  - #4   Bone Conduction Implant
    - BAHA
    - Ponto
    - BoneBridge

The chart below compares attributes of the individual treatment options above:

COMPARE	Canal	Canal + HA	VSB	BC
Hear Sound	+	+	+	+
Localize Sound	+	+	+	X
Hearing In Noise	+	+	+	X
Infection	+	X	+	XXX
Cost Over Life	+	X	XX	XXX
Breakage	+	X	XX	XXX
Complexity	++	++	+++	+

Red "X" is negative and "+" is a positive attribute for each condition.

International Conferences

Multiple times each year, the professionals at Global Hearing travel around the world to host conferences in various international locations to offer advice and evaluation for patients and their families. Patients who choose to have treatment with us then travel to our facility in California for surgery and postoperative care.

We do not do surgery in other countries. The postoperative care is so critical to success, it would be a bad idea to do surgery and leave patients in the care of local medical professionals who are not experienced in our techniques and methods.

The upcoming conference schedule—to date having including countries such as Russia, China, Korea, Mexico, South America, and Europe—is available at www.atresiarepair.com. You can also register for these conferences at the same link.

Some patients or parents choose to travel to our facility for surgical treatment. For ear canal surgery, we ask you to stay for a three- or four-week period after surgery. For CAM repair, we request a four-week stay. Other, more minor procedures require less time in California for healing.

After these amounts of time, the ear canal and eardrum (and outer ear in the case of CAM) are sufficiently healed (usually about 90%) to be able to travel and fly safely. The risk of most complications has passed at that point as well.

Upon returning home we ask you to follow a schedule to send us updates including images taken with your mobile phone. We send a bag of medications home with you in case a complication arises that we need to treat. Many times, the medicine needed to treat certain complications may not be available in the patient's home country, so it's better to have it and not use it than to need it and not be able to find it!

Remote Consultation

On a regular basis, I have remote consultations with patients around the world using online video conferencing. Prior to these consultations, I must receive the patient's CT scan (performed at a minimum of 2.5 years of age or older) and an audiogram within the past one month so that I can review the tests and determine surgical candidacy. The remote consultation then gives me an opportunity to discuss my findings and suggestions with families personally, and to help them develop an individualized treatment plan. Many families from our conferences around the world send data to our office after consultation at a conference for review and grading via HEAR MAPS score.

The following items are ideal for us to determine your child's HEAR MAPS score:

- A recent audiogram performed on both ears (whether affected or not affected). This can be emailed to our office or mailed to us along with the following items:
- Photos of the patient from four angles: front, right, and left, and from below the chin looking up, as well as close-up images of the affected ear.
- A temporal bone CT scan (your child should be at least 2.5 years of age for the CT). This entails having the scan performed, getting the images printed onto a CD, and mailing the disc to our office prior to any consultation with us. If only the film sheets themselves are available, you can likewise mail these to our office. In some cases, online file sharing is possible. I prefer to have the original digital images so I can use customized software to model the inner and middle ears.

A complete listing of how to make an appointment and what is needed can be found on our website at www.atresiarepair.com.

In-Office Consultations

You are welcome to contact California Ear Institute (CEI) to make an in-person appointment at our office in California.

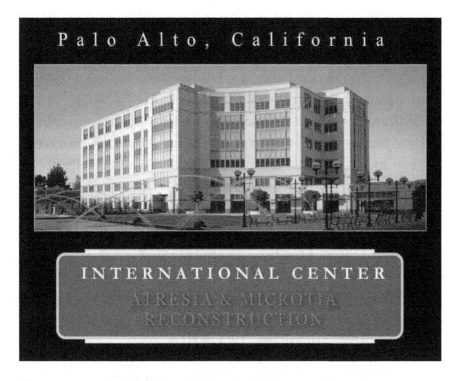

Our contact and mailing information is:

Global Hearing
The International Center for Atresia & Microtia Reconstruction
1900 University Avenue, Suite 101
East Palo Alto, CA 94303 USA

Phone 650-494-1000
(dial 011 first if calling from international numbers)
Email for appointments and inquiries:
atresiarepair@calear.com

Global Hearing and CEI

Why would people travel from around the world to California for CAAM surgery with Global Hearing? That is an excellent question for anyone investigating options to receive care for this condition.

Many surgeons around the world discourage surgery for CAAM. In our experience, however, extreme attention to detail, state-of-the-art equipment and facilities, and a dedicated world-class team can and do produce excellent, long-lasting results *in properly selected patients*. Surgeons need to know when to say no to trying to surgically create an ear canal—and when to use an alternate strategy to get hearing to an ear.

Through a rich and long history in the treatment of CAAM, Global Hearing has pioneered several techniques and strategies that translate to improved results for patients. These include the following:

Three New Surgeries for CAAM

- Canal surgery before microtia surgery
- Micro-incision canal surgery
- CAM repair in a single surgery

Complication Reduction:

- Reduction of stenosis incidence to under 2%
- Reduction in the displacement of the ear-drum to under 3%
- Reduced scarring, faster healing, and reduced pain with a skin graft
- Reduced skin problems of the ear canal using Angel Graft technique

Middle Ear Bone Reconstruction

- First to recognize fibrous IS joint in CAAM patients in 27% of cases

---

It is our experience that nearly every ear can hear. The question is how to achieve that goal for each child.

CEI is an internationally known center of excellence for the treatment of ear disease. Founded in 1968, CEI has become a treatment resource for tens of thousands of patients, with its rich heritage of state-of-the-art treatments and surgeons. In addition, the Institute has been fertile ground for advancements in ear disorder treatment, with several surgical procedures, several companies, and many new implantable devices that have come from its talented staff of physicians and scientists.

Providers at CEI focus solely on one area of expertise, including audiology and hearing devices, cochlear implants, craniofacial disorders, maxillofacial issues, sinus disease, sleep apnea, and plastic surgery. Located in Silicon Valley adjacent to Stanford University, CEI enjoys a rich and rewarding practice in a gorgeous environment.

www.ceimedicalgroup.com
www.letthemhear.org

We feel privileged and blessed to have received the trust of so many patients with CAAM. When I think of what my own children mean to me, I realize there may be no higher compliment than a parent putting trust in someone to operate on and care for their child. Treatment is still improving, and we will continue to strive for better and better outcomes as we tackle CAAM. Thank you to all who have allowed us to treat their family!

Chapter 6

Other Resources

Several repositories of information exist with resources available for you to explore. We have spent a significant amount of time and energy on our website, which contains more information for your use. Patients who are scheduled for surgery or who have had surgery previously will find sections giving instructions for both surgery preparation and postoperative care. Should you schedule surgery with us, you will receive all appointment times and information via email prior to your visit to our facilities. Many people find the FAQ section of our website helpful for exploring general questions and investigating unique and unusual situations that might pertain to you or your child.

Website: www.atresiarepair.com

Social media platforms can be fantastic to learn more as well, and we actively support the following:

 @ atresiarepair

 www.facebook.com/atresiarepair

Evaluation Summary Timeline

At Birth:
- **Hearing testing** of both ears (whether or not they are affected by CAAM!) as soon as possible following birth; complete all normal **newborn screening** testing as recommended by your birth center
- **Soft Band BCHA** fitting as early as possible in life, preferably <6 months old (mandatory in bilateral CAAM, optional in unilateral CAAM)

0 – 2.5 Years:
- Put together your care team:
    - **Pediatrician** – general physical examination, routine check-ups, immunizations, treat any ear infections in non-CAAM ear (if applicable), genetic testing a applicable, test for syndromes (if applicable)
    - **Audiologist** – establish care and monitor hearing, fit with BCHA device if needed; preferably pediatric audiologist familiar with hearing testing in children
    - **Otologist** – contact to establish care, begin filling in HEAR MAPS acronym evaluation system

- o **Plastic Surgeon** – select outer ear reconstructive method by 2.5 years of age, and contact plastic surgeon of your choosing to establish care
- o **± Craniofacial Surgeon** – if evaluation or treatment is needed for jaw and/or facial reconstruction
- At approximately 1 year of age, consult with **speech pathologist** if available to ensure speech & language skills are age-appropriate
  - o Continue with regular **speech & language therapy** if recommended by speech pathologist
- Consider attending one of GHI's international **Atresia Microtia Conferences** for an in-person consultation with our team
- Address any other medical conditions (cardiac, etc.) that must be treated prior to elective ear surgery

2.5 Years:
- Complete diagnostic testing
  - o **Temporal Bone CT Scan** – performed no earlier than 2.5 years of age
  - o **New Audiogram** – including air and bone conduction levels for both ears (whether or not they are affected by CAAM!)
- Send diagnostic testing to otologist for evaluation and treatment plan
- Select treatment plan and schedule surgery

Affected Ear/s:
Right
Left
Bilateral

HEAR MAPS Score: (Right / Left) Ear
H__.__ E___ A___ R___ M___ A___ P___ S___

Hearing
Bone Conduction/Nerve Function: _____
Air Conduction: _____

External Ear
Grade 1 / 2 / 3 / 4

Atresia Score — CT
1–10: _____
Complete Atresia / Partial Canal

Remnant Lobe
Normal
Reduced
Absent
Displaced

Mandible
Normal
Mild reduced
Moderate reduced
Severe reduced

Asymmetry of facial soft tissue
Normal
Mild reduced
Moderate reduced
Severe reduced

Paralysis of facial nerve
Normal
Mild reduced
Moderately reduced
Severe reduced
No movement, normal muscle tone
No movement, poor muscle tone

Syndromes
None identified to date
Other: _____

Associated Conditions
None
Yes: _____
Partial ear canal
Bilateral CAAM
Cholesteatoma
Fibrous IS joint
Hemi-facial microsomia/facial asymmetry
Jaw abnormalities & correction
Ear infections
PET's
Tonsil and adenoid enlargement
Sleep Apnea

Evaluation Summary Timeline

HEAR MAPS Score: (Right / Left) Ear

H__.__ E__ A__ R__ M__ A__ P__ S__

Hearing
Bone Conduction/Nerve Function: ____
Air Conduction: ____

External Ear
Grade 1 / 2 / 3 / 4

Atresia Score — CT
1–10: ____
Complete Atresia / Partial Canal

Remnant Lobe
Normal
Reduced
Absent
Displaced

Mandible
Normal
Mild reduced
Moderate reduced
Severe reduced

Asymmetry of facial soft tissue
Normal
Mild reduced
Moderate reduced
Severe reduced

Paralysis of facial nerve
Normal
Mild reduced
Moderately reduced
Severe reduced
No movement, normal muscle tone
No movement, poor muscle tone

Syndromes
None identified to date
Other: _____

Associated Conditions
None
Yes: _____
Partial ear canal
Bilateral CAAM
Cholesteatoma
Fibrous IS joint
Hemi-facial microsomia/facial asymmetry
Jaw abnormalities & correction
Ear infections
PET's
Tonsil and adenoid enlargement
Sleep Apnea

About Dr. Joe Roberson

At the start of his career, Dr. Joseph B. Roberson, Jr., MD served as the Director of Otology-Neurotology of the Skull Base Surgery Program at Stanford University. During his 10 years at the university, he focused on hearing-related brain tumors and cochlear implants as well as a small number of CAAM patients. Since 2004, he has served as Chief Executive of the California Ear Institute Medical Group and its many related medical entities.

In the 1990s, there was still a great deal of room for improvement in the treatment of CAAM, and the need for a center of excellence for the condition. Dr. Roberson began to focus on CAAM and established the International Center for Atresia & Microtia Repair and Global Hearing to respond to this need and to focus on this condition with a goal of improving results.

In 2002, Dr. Roberson and his wife started The Let Them Hear Foundation, a non-profit Christian organization that helps treat deafness in children and adults. Since then, the foundation has provided assistance to set up multiple cochlear implant programs around the world, including training surgeons and staff. More than 100 Surgeons have been trained through this program while Dr. Roberson has performed more than 100 cochlear implants in international venues personally. Due to the programs LTHF initiated, more than 5,000 deaf children in countries around the world have received the gift of hearing through a cochlear implant.

At this time, Dr. Roberson's main focus is the surgical care of children and adults with CAAM. He has treated over 3,000 patients from over 55 counties around the world. He still cares for many patients with a wide variety of ear- and skull-related disorders.

A Personal Note from Dr. Roberson

I like difficult problems, especially if they involve a situation in the operating room and they deal with issues children face—and even more if others don't do them well and there is an opportunity to improve results. In my opinion, the surgical correction of CAAM is the hardest challenge ear surgeons face. It's so difficult, in fact, that many ear surgeons do not even recommend surgery.

During the early part of my career (in addition to CAAM), I focused on refining the process of cochlear implantation and surgery for a type of brain tumor called an acoustic neuroma (vestibular schwannoma) while serving as the Director of the Otology-Neurotology and Skull Base Surgery Program at Stanford University. I enjoyed teaching young trainee surgeons for just under a decade during my tenure at the university and have continued to train surgeons here at CEI who have finished prior training at numerous prestigious otolaryngology training programs. As the year 2000 approached, I was drawn more and more to CAAM. I think, in part, this was because improved surgical techniques had been successfully developed for each of the areas of my early focus, and now could be treated with excellent results that many surgeons are capable of providing. It was my desire to produce the same excellent outcomes for CAAM and to develop the procedures to make this possible.

We like to think we had a part in the overall progress of developing treatment of many of the conditions I specialized in early in my career. For example, through the Let Them Hear Foundation, numerous cochlear implant programs have been established internationally, where local surgeons and staff in international sites can receive training in treating certain types of deafness. The foundation has helped spread the expertise to implant these miraculous devices that can treat deafness in both children and adults. We have been, and continue to be, privileged to provide hearing both directly and indirectly to thousands of deaf children as a result (see www.lethemhear.org for more information). Another book I have written details a parent's decisions in the treatment of sensorineural deafness using cochlear implants and encapsulates many of the areas I participated in developing in this period of my career (in *Hear for Life: Dr. Joe's Guide to Your Child's Hearing Loss*). A third publication deals with some miraculous and remarkable stories that have resulted from our LTHF activities (in *Let Them Hear: An Ear Surgeon's Joyful Experience with Enabling People to Hear for the First Time*).

In the early 2000s, I began to focus on treating CAAM even more, with the hopes of achieving the same results and surgical advances in treatment. I now travel to multiple international countries each year to host conferences for parents and children affected by CAAM. In 2003, I founded the California Ear Institute Medical Group, which expanded CEI, originally founded in 1968. Moving into the non-university-affiliated healthcare environment has allowed better development and focus on CAAM and its treatment. Since 2004, when CEI and associated entities became a separate organization, I have been privileged to operate on patients from more than 55 countries with this condition.

CAAM is rare, which means few doctors have significant experience with its treatment. That fact also leads to something we see far too often: doctors who mean well (but who don't actually know a lot about CAAM) frequently give misleading or wrong advice to parents. They don't mean to harm, of course, but parents must avoid the mistake of thinking all advice received from a physician is correct. Since you are reading this book, you have already started the process of getting accurate and up-to-date information—good job!

The need for a center of excellence for CAAM was obvious, as the results we saw in the treatment of CAAM in the 1990s needed improvement. It was a challenge I accepted. Having a center capable of making all aspects of treatment available is the best way I know of to focus on new and innovative solutions—something we are proud to have achieved in the last two decades. Our physicians see a large volume of this condition and can collaborate freely to maximize outcomes as a result. As you have seen in the text, several disciplines are needed to evaluate and treat this condition. All those individuals are brought together under one roof at the International Center for Atresia & Microtia Repair at the CEI Medical Group. I hope you get to meet them—they are incredible. I owe so much to the staff, care providers, physicians, and surgeons at CEIMG who work so diligently to advance this art and science! We believe there is no greater honor, calling, responsibility, or privilege than to be entrusted with the care of children with CAAM—and perhaps, your own child. This is the highest compliment you can give us, and we are overwhelmingly grateful for that trust.

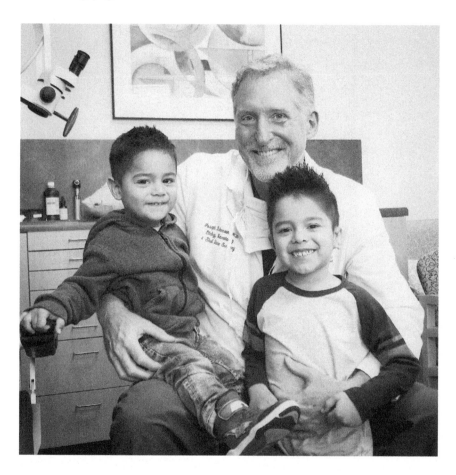

Endnotes

[1] Roberson, J. B., Reinisch, J., Colen, T. Y., & Lewin, S. (2009). Atresia repair before microtia reconstruction: comparison of early with standard surgical timing. *Otology & Neurotology : Official Publication of the American Otological Society, American Neurotology Society [and] European Academy of Otology and Neurotology, 30*(6), 771–776.

[2] Kaplan, A. B., Kozin, E. D., Remenschneider, A., Eftekhari, K., Jung, D. H., Polley, D. B., & Lee, D. J. (2016). Amblyaudia: Review of Pathophysiology, Clinical Presentation, and Treatment of a New Diagnosis. *Ymhn, 154*(2), 247–255.

[3] Lieu, J. E. C., Tye-Murray, N., Karzon, R. K., & Piccirillo, J. F. (2010). Unilateral Hearing Loss Is Associated With Worse Speech-Language Scores in Children. *Pediatrics, 125*(6), e1348–e1355.

[4] Roberson, J. B., Jr, Goldsztein, H., Balaker, A., Schendel, S. A., & Reinisch, J. F. (2013). International Journal of Pediatric Otorhinolaryngology. *International Journal of Pediatric Otorhinolaryngology, 77*(9), 1551–1554.

[5] R.A. Jahrsdoerfer, J.W. Yeakley, E.A. Aguilar, R.R. Cole, L.C. Gray, Grading system for the selection of patients with congenital aural atresia, Am. J. Otol. 13 (1992) 6–12.

[6] Goldsztein, H., & Roberson, J. B. (2013). Anatomical Facial Nerve Findings in 209 Consecutive Atresia Cases. *Otolaryngology--Head and Neck Surgery : Official Journal of American Academy of Otolaryngology-Head and Neck Surgery*, 1–5.

[7] Goldsztein, H., Ort, S., Roberson, J. B., Jr, & Reinisch, J. (2012). Scalp as split thickness skin graft donor site for congenital atresia repair. *The Laryngoscope*, pp. 1-3.

[8] Roberson, J. B. Combined Atresia Microtia (CAM) Repair – a new technique for reconstruction of form and function in congenital atresia and microtia. In Press, Microtia Repair. Editors Reinisch J, Tahiri Y.

[9] Anthropomorphic growth study of the head. Cleft Palate Craniofac J, 1992 vol. 29(4) pp. 303-308.

[10] Service, G. J., & Roberson, J. B. (2010). Alternative placement of the floating mass transducer in implanting the MED-EL Vibrant Soundbridge. *Operative Techniques in Otolaryngology-Head and Neck Surgery, 21(3),* 194–196.

[11] Balaker, A. E., Roberson, J. B., & Goldsztein, H. (2014). Fibrous Incudostapedial Joint in Congenital Aural Atresia. *Otolaryngology--Head and Neck Surgery : Official Journal of American Academy of Otolaryngology-Head and Neck Surgery.*